THE HEART TRUTH

DR AASHISH CONTRACTOR

THE HEART TRUTH

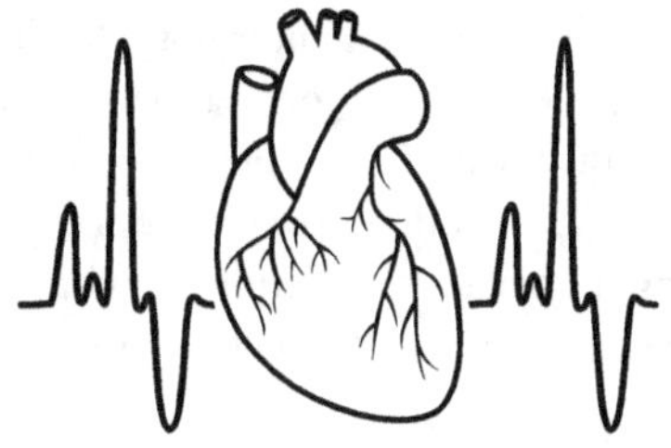

EVERYTHING YOU WANTED TO KNOW
ABOUT PREVENTION, TREATMENT
AND REVERSAL OF HEART DISEASE

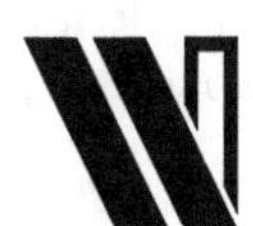

First published by westland ltd in 2016

Published by Westland Books, a division of Nasadiya Technologies Private Limited, in 2024

No. 269/2B, First Floor, 'Irai Arul', Vimalraj Street, Nethaji Nagar, Alapakkam Main Road, Maduravoyal, Chennai 600095

Westland and the Westland logo are the trademarks of Nasadiya Technologies Private Limited, or its affiliates.

ISBN: 9789360454876

10 9 8 7 6 5 4 3 2 1

Typeset in Adobe Garamond Pro by SÜRYA, New Delhi
Printed at Nutech Print Services, India

Contents

CONTENTS

Foreword

I AM MOST GRATEFUL TO DR AASHISH CONTRACTOR FOR WRITING THE BOOK *The Hearth Truth* when our country is witnessing an 'epidemic' of premature coronary artery disease.

Yes, unlike the popular perception, coronary artery disease is not a disease of old, retired people, it is a disease of young breadwinners of the family. In my practice, it is not the young man escorting his old father for the bypass surgery, it is the old father accompanying his young son for the bypass.

Dr Contractor has also clearly elucidated that bypass or angioplasty is not a cure, it is just the beginning of a long journey to prevent progression of the disease. He has, in this wonderful book, done what we should have as surgeons and cardiologists to every patient we treat. Easily understandable by a layman, every Indian must read the book if they want to celebrate their ninetieth birthday upright rather than on a wheelchair.

Dr Devi Shetty
Cardiac surgeon, founder and chairman of Narayana Health

Prologue

At 11:16 a.m., on 15 January 2012, Dhananjay Yellurkar crossed the finish line of the Standard Chartered Mumbai Marathon at CST station, 5 hours and 36 minutes after he had started from the same spot. After running for 42.2 km, he still managed to lift both arms in a victory salute, though the rest of his body was ready to shut down. As he stumbled past the mass of people who had gathered to witness celebrities finish the Dream Run (6 km), a large number of reporters surrounded him. They started peppering him with questions on his run and his emotions after having completed the full marathon.

The rule of thumb in Mumbai is that if 10 people surround a person and seem interested in him then, like moths to a flame, 50 more will gather in seconds. One of the 50 turned to me quite bewildered and asked what the fuss was all about. '*Kaun hai yeh?*' were his exact words, since Dhananjay wasn't a Bollywood celebrity, a politician, or even a TV star. He was a slightly-built 48-year-old banker, who looked just like any other Mumbaikar. Just then, he removed his sweat-drenched t-shirt and the secret of his 'celebrity-hood' was revealed. There was a long vertical scar running across his chest, where it had once been cut open to perform a heart bypass surgery. Dhananjay was a warrior who had stared heart disease and death in the face and come back to not only survive, but also achieve marathon glory.

After the media interaction, he walked up to the medical tent, where he was greeted with rousing cheers from several other 'patients' (I hate to use that word, since they are healthier than most 'normal' people in our city) with heart disease, who had also completed the run. Out of the 100 patients I had trained, 25 of them had completed the half marathon, and 75 had run the Dream Run. This was truly a celebration from the heart and watching it unfold got me thinking of that much used and abused phrase, 'reversal of heart disease'. If there ever was a group of people who had conquered heart disease, it was these bravehearts.

There is a huge volume of literature written on the subject of prevention and reversal of heart disease, and there are many theories on how to do it, ranging from the scientific to the outright bizarre. Is there one 'best method'? A method that is sustainable and yet effective? This question got me thinking and, after months of poring through all the information available, I arrived at the answer. In this book, I have combined this information along with my experience of the last 18 years and treating more than ten thousand patients. Over the next 21 chapters, I intend to take you on a journey through the heart, and empower you with the knowledge needed to prevent and reverse heart disease. Life is a journey, not a destination, so I hope you enjoy the journey as much as I enjoyed writing it.

1

Working of the Heart

(Three billion heart beats)

NO OTHER ORGAN IN THE BODY HAS RECEIVED AS MUCH ATTENTION over the centuries as the heart. It is considered the seat of all human emotions and has been most closely associated with love. It is also associated with bravery: think of Richard the Lionheart, or the oft-used expression 'braveheart'. The heart is also linked with kindness, as in, 'He has a kind heart', or the opposite of it, 'He is so heartless'. It's also considered to be a bag in which we put our feelings. We often talk about a person's heart being filled with joy or sorrow and many other emotions.

No wonder then that ailments of the heart attract so much more attention than any other part of our body. At the centre of all this attention is a small organ, no larger than the size of your fist. Its sole function is to act as a pumping station, which receives and distributes blood. It would not be wrong to say that, in terms of function, it's far less complicated than most organs in our body, such as our brain, kidneys and liver. Yet, in terms of importance, it occupies centre space. How often have you heard someone say, 'She fell in love and gave him her brain,' or someone being called a 'bravekidney', or someone's liver being filled with joy?

Home is where the heart is

They say that home is where the heart is. To easily understand the functioning of the heart, think of it as a house. This house has two rooms on the ground floor and two more above it. The lower two rooms, or chambers, are called ventricles, and the upper two chambers are called atria (the singular is 'atrium'). The upper and lower chambers are separated by a door on each side. These doors are called valves, and open only in one direction. The left and right side of the heart are divided by a wall in between, thus forming a left and right atrium, and a left and right ventricle. The heart lies in the chest cavity, slightly towards the left, and is protected by your breast bone, known as the sternum. It narrows towards the bottom and is angled to the left.

Flow of blood

Blood is transported from the upper and lower part of your body to the heart through blood vessels (veins), known as the superior and inferior venacava respectively. They enter the heart through the right atrium. This blood is collected from various organs of the body, after the oxygen in it has been consumed. It's therefore deoxygenated, and commonly referred to as 'impure blood'. The blood then flows down to the right ventricle, after passing a set of valves. From the right ventricle, this impure blood is carried to the lungs via the pulmonary arteries. Remember, the pulmonary arteries are the only arteries to carry impure blood in the body. In the lungs, oxygen from the air we breathe is exchanged for carbon dioxide, and oxygenated (pure) blood is transported to the left atrium of the heart via the pulmonary veins (the only veins to carry pure blood). From the left atrium, blood travels to the left ventricle after passing through the mitral valve. From the left ventricle, blood is pumped to the entire body, via the aorta, the largest artery in our body.

Your heart works as a muscular pump

The simplest way to describe the working of the heart is as a muscular pump. In order to fulfil its function, the heart needs to contract (to pump blood) and relax (to allow blood to fill) in a rhythmical manner. The heart muscle, which is vital for its functioning, is known as the myocardium. The contraction of the heart is known as systole (pronounced sys-toe-lee), and relaxation is called diastole (pronounced die-as-toe-lee). Each time the heart contracts, it's counted as a heart beat, and the number of times the heart beats in a minute is known as the heart rate. As the section below explains, you can easily measure your heart rate, commonly known as your pulse.

People often ask what their normal pulse or heart rate should be, and in school we were taught, 72 beats per minute. I'm not sure why all the biology texts have hit upon that number, but a normal heart rate can be anywhere between 60-100 beats per minute. A heart rate below 60 is known as bradycardia, and above 100 is known as tachycardia. Usually, most people have a heart rate somewhere between 65-85 beats per minute. Often, athletes and very fit sportspersons have heart rates that are well below 60, and it has been said that some super-athletes have heart rates below 40 beats/minute. When you exercise, your heart rate is supposed to increase, so do not measure your heart rate during or immediately after exercise, and confuse it with your resting heart rate. So, at what level of resting heart rate should you be concerned? Actually, there is no pre-defined level below or above which one must consult a doctor, but I would suggest getting it checked if it is consistently below 55 beats/minute (and you are not a super-athlete) or above 100 beats/minute at rest.

How to measure your pulse

If you want to measure your resting heart rate (pulse), make sure you are truly resting when you take it. A good time to measure it is just after you wake up, and are still in bed. You may not remember to do it then, so any other time is fine, but do not take it immediately after a period of exertion or excitation. Follow these simple steps:

1. Face the palm of any one of your hands upward and place three fingers (index, middle, and ring finger) of the other hand at the base of the thumb, slightly below the crease on your wrist. At this location your fingers will be resting on your radial artery. It's known as the radial artery since it runs along the radius bone of your forearm.
2. Move the fingers slightly till you feel the pulsation of your radial artery. If you are not able to locate it easily, apply gentle pressure and search again.
3. Once you find it, count the number of beats for a full minute, which is your heart rate.

4. You can also measure it at the side of your neck, in the hollow between
    your windpipe and the large muscle on the side. This is known as the
    carotid pulse, and you can use your index and middle finger to locate
    it, with very gentle pressure. This can be checked on either side of your
    neck, but make sure you don't check on both sides simultaneously, or
    very soon you won't have a pulse remaining!

The heart too needs blood

If we assume that your heart beats about 75 times per minute and you live
for 75 years, then in your lifetime your heart will have relaxed and contracted
3,000,000,000 times; that's three billion heart beats. Now that's a lot of work
even for the strongest braveheart! To provide energy for this mind-boggling
task, the heart muscle needs a constant supply of oxygen-filled blood. This
is supplied through blood vessels known as coronary arteries. These arteries
arise from the aorta soon after its exit from the left ventricle. They are called
the right and left main coronary artery. The left further divides into the left
anterior descending artery (LAD) and the left circumflex artery. They run on
the outer surface of the heart. An easy way to visualize it is to look at your
clenched fist. You will notice some blood vessels running on the outer surface,
which are very similar to the way your coronary arteries travel on the surface
of your heart. Just as your house has pipes supplying it with water, which is
essential for the survival of the household, these arteries supply blood to the
heart for its survival. (The only difference being that the coronary arteries
always receive adequate supply, unlike the water pipes in your house which
are dependent on the local municipality!)

Take-home messages

- The heart is a muscular pump, which supplies blood to the whole body.

- Think of the heart as a house, with four chambers; the upper two are called atria, and the lower two are called ventricles.

- Resting heart rate (pulse) is usually between 65-85 beats per minute.

- For the heart to function, it needs its own blood supply, which comes from three coronary arteries and their branches: left anterior descending artery, left circumflex artery and right coronary artery.

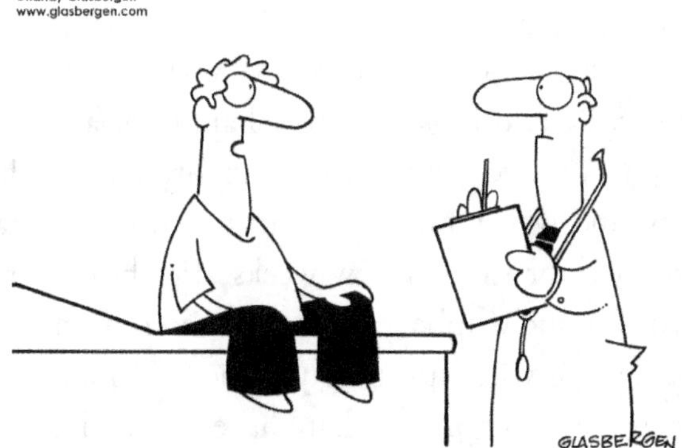

"I already diagnosed myself on the Internet.
I'm only here for a second opinion."

2

Problems of the Heart

(Heartaches and heart breaks)

THE FIRST TIME I MET MR RAMESH THAWANI AFTER HIS BYPASS SURGERY, he was with his wife and looking rather happy for a person who had just been operated on. A 58-year-old garment exporter, Ramesh clearly had a type-A personality, and was itching to return to work. Normally patients look quite apprehensive for the first few weeks after heart surgery, but in this case, he seemed extremely upbeat. When I asked him the reason for his happiness, he looked at his wife and smugly replied, 'For all these years, she said I had no heart, and now it's proven that I have one, and it had to be fixed because of the worries she caused me.' I did not want to enter a minefield of marital issues, so I deftly changed the subject, but as you can see, the heart can face many different types of problems.

Trouble in the house

As discussed in the earlier chapter, think of the heart as a house, and then it becomes easy to understand the various ailments that plague it. Just as a house can have structural, mechanical, electrical and plumbing problems, so can the heart. In this chapter, we will touch upon all of these, but it's important to keep in mind that the 'plumbing' problems of the heart are by far the most common. These are the blockages that take place inside the coronary arteries, leading to angina, heart attack, and even death. In medical terms, it is known as coronary heart disease or coronary artery disease.

Electrical problems

Each time your heart beats, or contracts, it does so in a synchronized manner, such that the atria and ventricles work in coordination. Electrical impulses are initiated in the right atrium, and spread through the heart in an organized manner. When the electrical impulses are transmitted haphazardly, you may feel uncomfortable beating sensations in your chest, which we commonly refer to as palpitations. In medical terms, these are known as arrhythmias or abnormal heart rhythms. Depending on their frequency and nature they can be harmless, which most of them are, or they can be life-threatening. An advanced study of abnormal electrical conduction patterns in the heart is known as an EP—electrophysiological study—and is done by a cardiologist who has specialized training in this area. Just as a good electrician is hard to find for your house, trained electro-physiologists are always in short supply.

A pacemaker is often implanted to solve the rhythm problems of the heart. It's a small metal device, about the size of half your palm, and is inserted under the skin, just below the collarbone on either side of your chest. A wire, known as a lead, runs from the machine to your heart chamber, and this helps control the electrical activity of the heart in a synchronized manner.

Mechanical problems

The heart has valves inside it which permit the flow of blood in one direction only. The most important valves are the mitral valve, which lies between the left atrium and ventricle, and the aortic valve, which lies at the entrance of the aorta. It is possible that, over time, the valves may either get too stiff or too loose. If they are too stiff, they will not open freely (a condition known as stenosis), and this hampers the flow of blood. On the other hand, if they are too loose (a condition known as regurgitation), they will flap back and allow the backflow of blood. In either of these conditions, adequate blood flow to the body will be compromised and the person may develop symptoms such as breathlessness. If the stenosis or regurgitation is severe, the valve may need to be surgically repaired or replaced.

Structural problems

The human heart is one of the first organs that is developed in the foetus—it begins forming within the first four weeks of pregnancy. It is usually fully formed within seven weeks. In rare instances, during formation, there may be abnormalities in the structure of the heart. These may manifest soon after birth, or sometimes remain undetected for several years. They are called congenital defects and the most common one is a hole in the heart. In a normal heart, the right and left chambers are separated by a wall, so that the impure and pure blood do not mix. When there is a structural defect (opening) in the wall, it is referred to as a hole in the heart. This allows impure blood to enter the aorta, and get pumped to the rest of the body. Mixing of pure and impure blood gives a bluish tinge to the skin, and hence the term 'blue baby' is sometimes used to describe congenital heart disease. Depending on the size of the opening, it may need to be operated to close it or may be left open and followed up with close medical supervision.

Plumbing problems

The heart pumps blood to the whole body for its survival, but at the same time, it needs to pump some of that blood back to itself for its own functioning. Coronary arteries run on the outer surface of the heart and supply blood to the heart muscle (myocardium) to allow it to pump efficiently. Blockages in the coronary arteries are what we conversationally refer to as heart disease. The more correct term would be 'coronary artery disease' (CAD), or 'coronary heart disease' (CHD). Due to these blockages, which are also known as plaques, the heart muscle receives inadequate blood supply, a condition known as ischemia. Therefore, coronary artery disease is also referred to as ischemic heart disease (IHD).

Heart disease is the largest cause of death in the world, both in men and women. The formation of this killer disease takes place over several years, and can therefore be halted if adequate preventive measures are taken in time. To understand how to prevent this from happening, or to reverse it once it has happened, we need to understand the process of atherosclerosis.

Process of atherosclerosis

The innermost lining of your coronary arteries are made up of living cells called the endothelium. These cells help in relaxing and contracting the arteries based on the requirement of blood by the heart muscle. Research has shown that the endothelium plays a vital role in the progression of atherosclerosis. Before we go further, I should explain the meaning of this tongue-twister. Its origin comes from the Greek words *athero*, which means gruel or paste, and *skleros*, which means hard. In other words, it's the hardening of the arteries due to the accumulation of plaque over time.

The process of atherosclerosis is initiated due to damage to the endothelium, which is caused by prolonged exposure to cardiovascular risk factors, such as elevated cholesterol, blood pressure, and smoking. You can think of the endothelium as the outer wall of a secure castle. Once that is breached and the enemy finds an opening, it's only a matter of time before it infiltrates inside and causes damage. In this case, the enemy is LDL or 'bad cholesterol', which enters the endothelium and gets deposited. The LDL molecules get oxidized in the presence of free radicals. Free radicals are not Naxalites roaming the jungles of central India, but are groups of atoms with an odd number of electrons. They are unstable and therefore 'steal' an electron from the LDL molecule to become stable, but in the process leave the LDL oxidized. The oxidized LDL is then engulfed by blood cells, and a series of reactions are set off, which lead to further build-up of plaque inside the artery. Inflammation also occurs at the site of plaque and recent research has been focused on the role of inflammation in heart disease.

You might have heard of antioxidants, which have been touted to have all sorts of wonderful healing properties against heart disease and cancer—one of their mechanisms of action is to prevent LDL being oxidized. The best known antioxidants are vitamins C, E, and beta carotene (a type of vitamin A). These act to neutralize the effects of free radicals in the body, and are most effective when consumed as part of a natural diet.

Table: Problems of the heart

Type of problem	Can lead to
Electrical	Palpitations – rhythm disturbances
Mechanical	Tight or loose valves
Structural	Hole in the heart
Plumbing	Blockages in the coronary arteries

Heart attack

The plaque is made up of cholesterol, calcium, dead materials from cells, and fibrin (clotting material present in the blood). Conventional thinking was that this plaque grew slowly over time, and ultimately became large enough to stop the flow of blood to the heart muscle and cause a heart attack. However, over the last couple of decades, we have learnt that at some point in its growth, the plaque cracks or ruptures, and that causes a large blood clot to be formed at the area of rupture. This blood clot, known as a thrombus, obstructs the flow of blood, leading ultimately to the death of a part of the heart muscle, known as myocardial infarction, or heart attack. Depending on the extent of damage to the heart muscle, the heart attack can be labelled as minor or major.

Size does not matter: 70 per cent blockage may be more dangerous than 100 per cent

When I met Mrs Anjali Sharma in cardiac rehabilitation, a month after her heart attack, she seemed quite upset. She said, 'Doctor, I just had an angiography two months ago, and my cardiologist told me that I had one blockage of 80 per cent and two more of about 50 per cent. An angioplasty was done for the bigger blockage, and I was told that I did not need any interventional procedure for the others. How could I have a heart attack with only a 50 per cent blockage?'

Unfortunately, Mrs Sharma's case is often the rule, rather than the exception. Research has shown that a majority of heart attacks occur due to blockages that are less than 70 per cent. The reason is plaque rupture, in which the extent of the artery blockage is not the crucial factor. In fact, that explains the paradox of why people can survive with even a 100 per cent blockage. It takes several years for an artery to be completely blocked (100 per cent), and often by that time, nature has provided an alternate blood supply through vessels known as collaterals. One of the primary aims of heart disease reversal is to facilitate the development of this collateral circulation. Also, since plaque rupture is the crucial step that leads to the heart attack, the goal of any prevention or reversal program is to stabilize the plaque to prevent it from rupturing.

©Randy Glasbergen www.glasbergen.com

GLASBERGEN

"My bones are getting softer, but my arteries
are getting harder, so it balances out!"

The perfect storm

In late 2012, a study was published which changed our understanding of how heart attacks occur. The study revealed that for an acute coronary event to occur (such as heart attack or death), multiple factors need to fall into place at the same time, leading to 'the perfect storm'. The factors and conditions associated with an increased risk for events include the composition and size of the plaque, blood clotting factors, hormonal influences, risk factors, and environmental factors such as pollution.

Plaques can be broadly classified into soft and hard. Soft plaques have a greater amount of cholesterol in them, and have a higher tendency to rupture and lead to a heart attack. Hard plaques have a lesser amount of cholesterol, but a higher amount of calcium and other substances, and are usually formed over a longer period of time. Soft plaques are more likely to rupture and are also called vulnerable plaque. Paradoxically, they cause less blockage of the coronary arteries and therefore often do not cause symptoms and are not picked up on routine tests.

Heart failure

Those of you who have grown up on Bollywood movies of the 1970s and '80s will recollect countless scenes where the doctor with a grim look on his face informs the hero about his father's condition and says, '*Unka* heart fail *ho gaya.*' By this, he usually means that the person has died, upon which the hero screams in anger and then weeps uncontrollably.

Somehow, this scene plays in my mind each time I need to inform a patient that they have heart failure. Since most of them have probably grown up on these same movies, I hasten to add that 'heart failure' is just a technical term, and it does not mean that their heart has stopped working or that they are going to die soon. Heart failure is a condition in which the amount of blood pumped out by the heart each minute is not enough to meet the needs of the body. This usually occurs when the heart muscle is weak and is unable to pump out sufficient blood. The commonest cause is coronary artery disease (with or without a heart attack). Other common causes are high blood pressure over a period of time and cardiomyopathy.

Patients with heart failure may be in a stable phase and live for a very long time, with no symptoms, while a few may go into an acute phase in which they feel extremely short of breath and may need to be hospitalized for a few days. Often the pumping capacity or ejection fraction of a heart failure patient is greatly reduced. During the relaxation phase of the heart cycle, the left ventricle fills with blood, which is pumped out during the contraction phase. However, all of the blood is not pumped out, and some remains inside the left ventricle. The percentage of blood pumped out is called the ejection fraction or EF. A normal EF is considered to be between 55–65 per cent, while in heart failure patients it can be as low as 15–20 per cent.

Cardiomyopathy

Another condition in which the heart muscle is weakened is cardiomyopathy. This is a disease of the heart muscle, in which the muscle becomes enlarged, thick or rigid. There are a variety of different cardiomyopathies, and the two most common ones are dilated cardiomyopathy and hypertrophic cardiomyopathy. The heart enlarges, but paradoxically becomes more inefficient in pumping blood. Think of the heart muscle becoming big and flabby, rather than big and strong (as happens with exercise). In many cases, the cause of this is unknown, though it is often genetic. Some of the known causes are long-term high blood pressure, a previous heart attack, and heart valve problems.

Many people with cardiomyopathy have no signs or symptoms, and the condition is picked up by chance on a routine echocardiogram. At the same time, there are others in whom the disease progresses very rapidly, with severe symptoms and complications. The symptoms are similar to those of heart failure, with shortness of breath being the predominant symptom.

Treatment of this condition varies from only medication to implantable devices, and some patients may even need a heart transplant.

The focus is on blockages

As you have seen by now, besides heartbreak the heart can suffer a plethora of problems from birth to death. However, do remember that when we talk about heart disease, we refer to the atherosclerotic plaques in the coronary arteries, which can also be called coronary heart disease, or coronary artery disease, or simply, blockages in the heart arteries. The rest of this book will focus on the prevention, reversal and treatment of these blockages, since it's by far the most frequently prevalent form of heart disease.

Take-home messages

- Problems of the heart can be broadly grouped into electrical (pacemaker), mechanical (valve), structural (hole in the heart) or plumbing (blockage).

- When we talk about heart disease, it usually refers to coronary heart disease, which is the formation of blockages in the coronary arteries.

- The process is called atherosclerosis and usually takes place over several years, due to deposition of cholesterol and other 'junk' substances in the inner lining of the coronary arteries.

- A heart attack (myocardial infarction) takes place due to a rupture in the blockage. The stability of the blockage matters more than the size, which is why a larger blockage is not necessarily more dangerous than a smaller one.

- Heart failure is a condition where the heart is not able to pump adequate blood to meet the demands of the body.

3

Tests to Detect Heart Disease

(How strong is your heart?)

AJEET ARENJA'S CT ANGIOGRAM REVEALED THAT HE HAD THREE BLOCKAGES in his heart arteries. However, all three of them were in non-critical locations and hence caused him no symptoms.

Mr Arenja is a jovial 60-year-old industrialist and my good friend Nithiij's father. I have known Nithiij well for the last 12 years, and have been his friend, philosopher and guide, especially in matters of medicine. Nithiij is one of those Google doctors, who look up medical conditions on the internet and come up with the diagnosis and treatment before any real doctor can. In the past he would come up with bizarre treatment options, all of which are available in plenty on the net. Then I taught him how to use Pubmed, the US government database of all articles published in medical journals. This is an act I sometimes regret, since he bombards me with several diagnoses for every medical problem, although I have to add that he also comes up with solutions, all of which have been published in reputed medical journals. And he is usually correct!

When his father turned 60, Nithiij insisted he undergo a full medical check-up which included a stress test. Mr Arenja passed all of these with flying colours, but then Nithiij insisted that he undergo a CT angiography just to be 'doubly' sure. Now that the CT angio revealed blockages, he had to go in for a 'regular' angiography to confirm the results. So, how did the case finally end? Let us have a look at all the testing options available for cardiac diagnosis, and we can then get back to his story.

History is important

All the tests described in this chapter are heart-specific tests which lead to the diagnosis of heart disease. But before doing any of these tests, it is crucial to study your full medical profile. This will help the doctor select which test is the most relevant for you. Do not underestimate the value of a good history. You need to describe your medical story in great detail, including any signs and symptoms you might have felt. Often an accurate diagnosis can be made with a good history, and the need for testing is reduced.

Which is the best test?

Doctors are used to having professional questions thrown at them in social settings. It usually starts with, 'Doc, I don't mean to bother you at a party, but I was just wondering if I could ask you one small question?' Depending on the person, and the social setting, that 'one small question' could be followed up by many more small questions, and you suddenly realize that you have conducted a full consultation in the host's living room over drinks and snacks.

I most frequently get asked about the best test to rule out the risk of getting a heart attack. And they want a 100 per cent surety!

The truth is that no single test exists which is foolproof. Each cardiac test will give you some information related to current or future risk, and all of it put together, along with a thorough medical history, will give you a good idea of your cardiac risk. Over the course of this chapter, I would like to discuss the most commonly performed cardiac tests and their strengths and weaknesses.

Electrocardiogram

Most people consider the electrocardiogram (ECG) to be a magical test which tells us all about the heart. While it is a very useful test, it does have its limitations, and that is sometimes hard for people to fathom. Patients and their family and, frankly, even doctors often wonder how a heart attack occurred, even when a recently taken ECG was normal.

As the name suggests, the electrocardiogram is a recording of the electrical activity of the heart. There are 10 'stickers', known as electrodes, put on various parts of your chest, wrists and ankles. These electrodes are connected by wires to the main unit. They look at your heart from 12 different angles, hence the term '12 lead ECG'. The activity is recorded as waves, which are the typical patterns you see on the special ECG paper, known as thermal paper. On this type of paper (which is heat sensitive), the recordings fade over time, and it's a good idea to take a photocopy of your ECG to preserve it for future reference.

Like a good, but not great astrologer, an ECG is able to fairly accurately give you an idea about your past history, but is not good at predicting the future. For example, it can show that you have had a heart attack in the past, but will not be able to indicate if you will have one in the next 10 minutes. To be fair to the ECG (and astrologers), it sometimes gives you clues of possible future problems, such as indications that some parts of the heart are not receiving adequate blood supply. If the person is in the midst of a heart attack (which can take several hours to evolve), an ECG can pick it up, and in such cases we repeat the test every few hours to track how the attack is progressing and the effect of medication on it.

An ECG is also good at picking up abnormal heart rhythms, such as extra heart beats or abnormally fast or slow heart beats. Therefore it would be right to say that it's an extremely important test which gives you information about the heart, but is by no means the only heart test that one should do. The interpretation of the ECG should be left to a trained doctor, who not only can read the ECG, but is also well aware of your clinical situation. In interpreting an ECG, especially one which seems to be abnormal, it's very helpful to have an older ECG to compare with. This allows the doctor to judge whether the changes seen are fresh and need urgent attention or are related to an older problem, which has been addressed. A word of caution here: do not look at the computerized diagnosis printed on your ECG. You will invariably read the phrase, 'Probably abnormal ECG', even if there is a minor aberration which has no clinical significance.

Echocardiogram

This test, which is commonly known as a 2-D (two dimensional) echo, uses the principle of ultrasound to study the functioning of the heart muscle and valves. A probe is moved over the left side of your chest, and sound waves are reflected off your heart chambers to form a visual representation of the same on the screen. This test is great at studying the functioning of the heart valves. It is not used specifically to detect blockages. However, abnormal movement of the heart muscle during the cardiac cycle can give an indication of inadequate blood supply, indicating blockages.

The 2-D echo is also good at calculating the ejection fraction (EF), which is commonly called the pumping capacity of the heart. One of my patients had a routine check-up a year after surgery and the results were excellent. However, when he met me his appearance suggested all was not well, which perplexed me. On digging deeper, he said, 'Doctor, my heart is not functioning properly.' This surprised me, since all his results were absolutely normal. He then said, 'My heart is beating only 60 per cent, so how can you say that's normal.' That's when it struck me that we often don't explain results carefully enough to patients. A normal EF is between 55–65 per cent, but it's natural for patients to assume that 100 per cent is normal, and therefore 60 is abnormal. There is no official categorization of the EF, but 45–55 per cent is considered slightly below normal, while 35–45 per cent is considered moderately below normal. If the EF is below 35 per cent, there is need for concern, but not panic. It's important to consult with your cardiologist, since it might indicate the presence of heart failure.

Stress test

Oftentimes, when patients are told that they need to undergo a stress test, they imagine it's some sort of mental test, which will put them under great stress. Actually, the test is done to put your heart under 'stress' and see how well it responds. A stress test is commonly referred to as a TMT, or treadmill test. A resting ECG is taken, after which you are made to exercise on a treadmill (or a stationary bike) using a fixed protocol. The Bruce protocol is most popular worldwide, in which the treadmill goes steeper and faster every three minutes. Your goal is to keep walking (or running) till you are fatigued and can go no further. This is very different from a regular exercise session on the treadmill, and is designed to fatigue you within 6 to 12 minutes. Patients often tell me, 'Doc, I can easily go for 30 minutes since I work out on the treadmill daily for that long.' I just smile at that, and remind them that even world-class athletes would not last more than 20 minutes on this protocol.

The purpose of the test is to compare your ECG at rest, versus that at maximum exercise to see if there are any changes. These changes, which are suggestive of reduced blood reaching your heart muscle, are indicative of blockages and are known as ST segment changes, or ST-T changes. An easy way to understand this concept is to think of water flow in your bathroom. When you need to wash your hands in your basin, you need a relatively small amount of water at a medium flow rate. But when you need to take a shower, there is a much greater need for both, amount of water and speed of flow. It's the same with your heart. At rest, your heart muscle needs only a small amount of blood flow. This need increases as you exercise and reaches

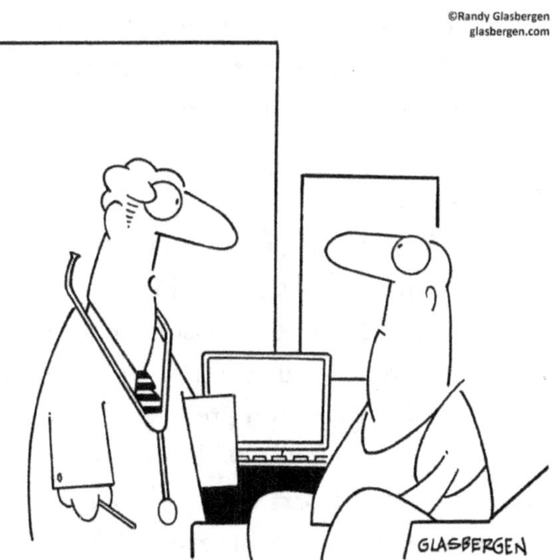

"Two hours in our waiting room with a bunch of coughing people and screaming children. That was your stress test."

its peak at your maximum exercise capacity. During the stress test, the doctor studies your ECG to see if there is a lack of blood supply to your heart muscle during exercise by comparing it to your resting ECG. In one of the many idiosyncrasies seen in medicine, an abnormal test is called a positive stress test and a normal test is termed negative.

A stress test is reasonably accurate, but sometimes fails to detect blockages even when they are present. This is because the test becomes positive (shows an abnormality) only when the blockages cross a certain size and obstruct the flow of blood. This usually happens when the blockages are 70 per cent or more in size. If you recall, in the previous chapter we spoke about how heart attacks can occur due to plaque rupture even when the blockages are smaller in size. This is one of the reasons why people sometimes have a heart attack even when their recent stress test is normal.

On the other hand, you sometimes have 'false positive' tests, which means that there isn't underlying atherosclerosis, though the test is abnormal. This is more commonly seen in women, and therefore doctors sometimes prescribe advanced stress tests such as stress thallium or stress echo for women.

Stress thallium and stress echo

Both of these tests have a greater degree of accuracy compared to a regular stress test. In a stress thallium, dye is injected in your veins and images are taken of your heart at rest and during exercise. The doctor studies how well the dye reaches various parts of your heart muscle and looks for areas of reduced dye uptake, which suggest compromised blood flow. The purpose of the test is to look for areas of 'reversible' and 'fixed' ischemia. A fixed defect or ischemia suggests that part of the heart muscle is not receiving blood either at rest or during exercise. Reversible ischemia suggests that the area is receiving blood during rest, and not during exercise. This has clinical significance, since the decision to carry out an intervention may be based on this information. Though a fixed defect would mean bad news, it also suggests that there is no point in doing a surgery or angioplasty in that area. After all, opening up the blood supply to that area would be akin to a gardener pouring water on a dead flower.

In a stress echo, the doctor performs a 2-D echo study of your heart before and immediately after exercise to look for changes in the contracting pattern of your heart muscle. The pattern of contraction is compared between rest and maximum exercise. If there is a compromise at both rest and exercise, then it's similar to the fixed defect described above. However, if the compromise is only during maximum exercise, then it's a reversible problem.

The key to any type of stress test is that it should ideally be done till maximum effort. You should be the one asking for the test to be stopped when you have reached your limit, unless the doctor sees some abnormality prior to that. Most centres around the country tend to stop the test at a predetermined predicted heart rate max, which often does not give the true picture.

After doing a stress test, patients often want to know if they have passed or failed the test, depending on how long they lasted on the treadmill. There really isn't any specific cut-off time to indicate that you have passed, but a general rule of thumb suggests that if you are below 60 years, you should be able to last at least eight to nine minutes on the test. Most of my patients who are training for the marathon comfortably cross 12 minutes on the test (and they have an unspoken internal competition to see who can cross 15 minutes!).

Stress tests are great indicators of cardiorespiratory fitness levels, and the amount of time a person is able to stay on the test also influences treatment decisions. For example, if a person gets mild ECG changes at 11 minutes on a Bruce protocol, we would approach the case very differently compared to changes seen at four minutes.

Angiography

This is considered the gold standard test to detect blockages in your coronary arteries. In this, a small incision is made in your groin, and a thin catheter is passed into the artery opening there, known as the femoral artery. Currently, the trend is shifting towards passing the catheter through the radial artery, by making a small incision in your wrist. The advantage of the radial approach is that you can be up on your feet almost as soon as the procedure is over, as compared with several hours of bed rest with the groin approach.

In both, the catheter is skilfully guided by the cardiologist through your arteries until it reaches the coronary arteries. Dye is injected into them and several images are taken at different angles, with the help of a rotating C-shaped machine. With the help of these images, the cardiologist can determine the location of the blockages as well as the extent to which they have blocked off the inside opening of the artery, known as the lumen. Therefore when the report says that it's 80 per cent stenosis (blockage), it means that the block has encroached upon 80 per cent of the free space inside the lumen.

The angiography is considered the gold standard, but it has its limitations. Scientists have shown that plaques also tend to grow outwards. When this happens the lumen is not encroached upon, or is minimally encroached upon, and does not give the true picture. The angiography is only able to detect 'inward' growth. Think of it as an iceberg below the water. What you see is only the tip outside the water. Similarly, the plaque could be growing silently outwards, within the walls of the artery, like a ticking time bomb, since it's undetected.

Also, an angiogram tells you about the presence of blockages, but it does not give you an idea about the nature of the plaque. As we had discussed in the previous chapter, soft plaques which are rich in cholesterol are more likely to rupture and cause a heart attack than hard ones.

To improve the diagnostic accuracy of the angiogram, and to help in making a decision regarding further course of action, a technique called fractional flow reserve, or FFR can be used. This measures the pressure difference in the flow of blood, on both sides of the blockage. Ideally, if the blockage is not obstructing flow, the ratio should be one. A ratio below 0.75–0.8 is considered abnormal and helps guide the further course of action.

CT angiography

At the same social events I referred to earlier, one of the most common questions asked is, 'Should I do a CT angiography?' My advice is against doing the test purely as a matter of routine. It should be done only when there are definite indications to perform the test.

In a CT angiography, a CT scan is taken of the heart and blood vessels and a 3-dimensional representation of the heart is created. As technology has improved, the correlation between the CT angio and the regular or catheter angio is very close to exact. However, when advanced tests like a CT scan are done without any clinical indications, they often show up results that can best be described as non-specific. So, even if we see mild atherosclerosis on the scan, we do not have enough evidence presently to show that treating it aggressively is any better than leaving it unattended. I usually recommend someone do the test when my judgment is leaning to the side of them having normal arteries, but the test is being done as a matter of abundant precaution. If, on the other hand, I think it's more likely that significant atherosclerosis is present, I would recommend a 'regular' angio.

Another aspect of CT scans that is rarely spoken about is the exposure to radiation. On an average, one cardiac CT scan could equal to 100–200 normal X-rays. This is an extremely high dose of radiation, and should not be done without appropriate reason. High radiation has been linked to an increased risk for future cancer. As technology progresses, some of the newer machines and techniques are able to reduce the amount of radiation, but it is still fairly high. Not just CT scans, even thallium tests lead to large radiation exposure and should not be done without adequate justification.

When should you test further?

The decision on when to test further and which is the best test to perform is often a judgment call on the part of your doctor. For example, if your stress test was positive, then the next step will depend on how 'abnormal' the test was. If the abnormal changes were seen at a very low level of exercise, and the changes were extensive, then it might make sense to go in for an angiography directly. On the other hand, if the changes were minor or took place at a very high level of exercise, it would be better to undergo a further 'functional' test such as a stress echo or stress thallium. If this functional test is abnormal, then an angio is the right choice, but if it is normal, then it's fine to observe and do no further testing.

Sometimes all tests may be normal, but you may have symptoms related to heart disease, such as chest discomfort. In such situations the decision-making becomes a lot harder.

Symptoms count

Usually, most people like to stay as far away from tests as possible, and would rest easy after a negative stress test. But that was not the case with Sunil Joshi. This 60-year-old Prabhadevi resident used to take a daily morning walk for several years. At one point he experienced mild abdominal discomfort during the walk, for which he diligently went and did a stress test. The test was negative after seven minutes on the treadmill, and he was told that all was well with his heart. He went back to his morning walks, but the uncomfortable sensation still remained. Mentally he knew that something was wrong, and he decided to go in for an angiography since his symptoms were persisting (even though his doctor said there was no need for further testing).

The angiography revealed four blockages and he underwent bypass surgery in January 2013. Unlike most patients, Sunil actually seemed proud of the fact that he had heart disease, because he had self-diagnosed it. He called himself a PhD in heart disease, and when asked to elaborate, said that he had high BP, which made him a graduate, he had diabetes which made him a double graduate, and his cholesterol was also high, so that got him the PhD degree. They say that laughter is the best medicine, and this description certainly had me in splits. Sunil was obviously enjoying himself and went on to point to his double chin, saying that he had a 'hereditary double *bandho*', which in Gujarati means he was fat. I have noticed that patients (and people in general) who have the ability to laugh at themselves always end up doing better, and Sunil Joshi was no exception.

As I have said earlier, no cardiac test is foolproof, and this was underscored in Sunil's example. The history that a patient gives is often the best guide to diagnosis and if a person is symptomatic, I would advise further testing, even if the initial test was clear. The flow chart below illustrates the decision-making process in different situations. Of course, it goes without saying that you must consult with your doctor when deciding on which test to do.

DECISION-MAKING PROCESS:WHICH TEST SHOULD YOU DO?

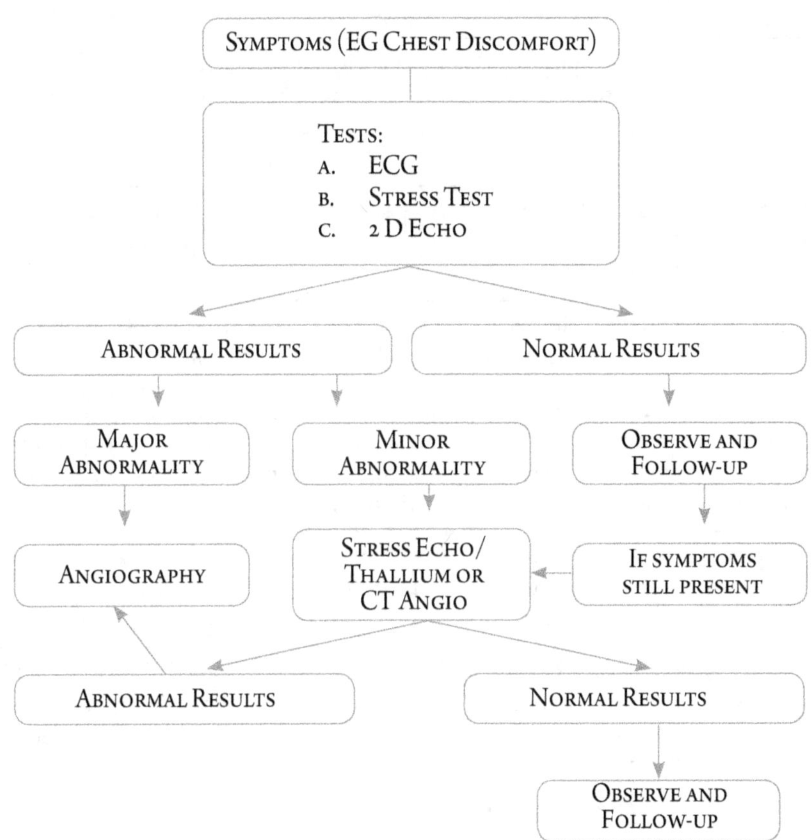

Pros and cons of commonly performed cardiac tests

Name of test	Primary use	Pros	Cons
ECG	To detect ongoing heart attack; to check for heart rhythm	Inexpensive and easy to administer	Normal ECG does not rule out blockages
2-D echo	To study heart valves and heart muscle functioning	Accurate and non-invasive	Dependent on 'operator'
Stress test	To detect blockages and assess cardiac fitness	Non-invasive	False-positive and false-negative tests do occur
Stress echo/ thallium	To detect blockages and assess cardiac fitness	Higher degree of accuracy compared to stress test	Radiation exposure (in stress thallium)
Angiography	To detect blockages in coronary arteries	Considered the gold standard test	Invasive and cannot detect blockages growing outwards
CT angiography	To detect blockages in coronary arteries	Non-invasive	Radiation exposure; if positive, follow-up angio usually needed too

Finally, which is the best test?

If you recollect, after Mr Arenja had a CT angio, he went in for a regular angiography which revealed similar blockages as the scan. As is quite common, he got conflicting opinions and at one point even booked a date for surgery. However, he did not have any symptoms and, after the angiography, was recommended to do a stress thallium study. He came to me for a second opinion, and wanted to know why a stress thallium was recommended after an angio, when it's usually the other way around.

Let me explain it this way: the angio is a test to see the anatomy of the artery. In other words, it looks at the structure of the artery, and whether there is plaque present. On the other hand, a stress thallium or any other type of stress test looks at the function or physiology of the artery and blood supply. As I had mentioned in the first chapter, think of the heart as a house that requires plumbing. Your arteries are like pipes which supply blood, instead of water. Now, if we had to study the inner lining of all our pipes which were probably laid in the times of British rule, we would find a lot of structural damage within. However, most of them still supply water in an adequate manner and there is no need to fix them. Similarly, there are often nasty-looking blockages inside the arteries, but if the blood supply to the heart muscle is not compromised, and the person is not symptomatic, then we can make a judgment call to not do anything to the blockage.

Mr Arenja did very well on his stress thallium and did not need surgery. I am happy to report that he is doing wonderfully well, under the watchful eye of 'doctor' Nithiij, who has him on an extremely disciplined lifestyle program.

So, we come back full circle from where we started this chapter, which is, there is no single best test to detect heart disease. The best test will depend on the specific information we seek, and usually a combination of tests will give us the full picture. The results of these tests need to be seen in context of the medical history. In addition to a good history, you need to measure risk factors for heart disease. These can be done by simple tests such as blood pressure measurement, blood tests for diabetes and cholesterol and weight and height measures. In the next chapter we will discuss each of these risk factors in detail.

Take-home messages

- There are a variety of tests used to detect heart disease, all of which give different information. There is no single test that can be labelled as best.

- The ECG is good at diagnosing heart attacks and rhythm disturbances.

- The 2-D echo is best to study the functioning of heart valves and the pumping capacity of the heart.

- A stress test looks at how the heart responds to stress (exercise), and helps detect blockages. Stress thallium and stress echo are more advanced stress tests.

- An angiography looks at the inside of the coronary arteries to detect blockages and their location. It looks at the anatomy (structure), while stress tests look at physiology (function). CT angiography gives you similar information done through a CT scan.

4

Risk Factors

(And how the heart is affected)

'YOU DOCTORS KEEP TELLING ME TO QUIT SMOKING, BUT JUST LOOK AT MY uncle Dinshaw. He smoked one packet a day, ate red meat and eggs daily and lived to the ripe old age of 92. And at the same time, look at Mahesh from my office—poor fellow had no vices, ate only boiled vegetarian food, lived like a sanyasi, walked 5 miles daily, and had a heart attack at 48.' This is the lecture I heard from a patient when I told him about all the lifestyle changes he needed to make to prevent a heart attack.

If I had a hundred rupees for every time I heard the above lines, or something very similar, I would be a very rich man. I usually hear it when I am trying to counsel someone to quit smoking, or take up exercise, or to eat healthy. There is truth in the statement that there are people who lead healthy lives and suffer from heart disease, and the other way around. However, to fully understand the reasons why this happens, we need to study why heart attacks occur in the first place.

What are risk factors?

Heart disease is caused due to the presence of 'risk factors'. Just as the term implies, a risk factor is any factor that increases the likelihood of disease. The easiest way to describe the impact of risk factors on heart disease is to compare it with driving a car. Imagine you are driving down Marine Drive in south Mumbai early on a Sunday morning at 30 kilometres per hour, with your car in perfect working condition. It would be fair to say that the chances of you having an accident are extremely slim. Now imagine speeding down that same road at 100 kilometres per hour. Clearly the odds of having an accident will increase slightly. What if your brakes were not working very well? Again, the chances of an accident will increase. What if you were driving after having a few drinks and it's raining heavily? Without doubt, in this scenario the chances of an accident are pretty high.

I would like you to consider two questions at this stage. First, is it possible (note the use of the word 'possible', and not 'likely') to have an accident in the scenario with conditions perfect for driving? Second, is it possible not to have an accident if you are driving fast, with bad brakes, heavy rain, and after a few drinks? Clearly, the answer to both questions is yes.

When driving a car, high speed, heavy rain, alcohol and bad brakes are all risk factors for having an accident. The greater the number of risk factors, the greater the chance of having an accident. However, there are a small percentage of cases when accidents occur even under perfect conditions, and sometimes people are plain lucky even under the worst conditions. It's exactly the same with heart disease. In other words, there are probably 5 per cent of people who lead risky lives, like Uncle Dinshaw, and do not have heart disease, and there are 5 per cent of people like Mahesh who have no risk factors, and still end up suffering. The important point here is that 90 per cent of the time, the eventual outcome will depend on how much care you have taken. So, unless you are prepared to risk your health on a gamble of 5 per cent, it makes sense to work hard on keeping your risk factors in check.

What are the risk factors for heart disease?

There are several strongly established risk factors which are known to cause heart disease, and new ones are being discovered every few years. On top of the list of known culprits is cigarette smoking and high blood pressure. Today it's a no-brainer that smoking is bad for your heart as well as a cause of several types of cancer, but this was not always the case. In fact, until the late 1950s, it was not considered harmful to smoke, and even the American Medical Association endorsed smoking as a healthful activity. So, then the question (especially one asked by tobacco companies) is, how do we know that smoking, or for that matter, cholesterol or high blood pressure is bad for your heart?

Most of the information that we have on this subject is derived from the Framingham Study (details below), which followed participants for years and studied those who eventually got heart attacks, and analyzed the reason for their heart attack.

The Framingham Heart Study

(Information taken from the official study website: www.framinghamheartstudy. org)

1. In 1948, the Framingham Heart Study was started in the United States with an objective to identify the common factors or characteristics that contribute to heart disease and stroke by following a large group of participants (for several decades) who had not suffered a heart attack or stroke at the start of the study.

2. The researchers enrolled 5,209 men and women between the ages of 30 and 62 from the town of Framingham, near the city of Boston, and began the first round of extensive physical examinations and lifestyle interviews that they would later analyze for common patterns related to heart disease development. Since 1948, the participants continued to return to the study every two years for a detailed medical history, physical examination, and laboratory tests. In 1971, the study enrolled a second-generation group—5,124 of the original participants' adult children and their spouses to participate in similar examinations.

3. Over the years, careful monitoring of the Framingham Study population has led to the identification of the major risk factors—high blood pressure, high blood cholesterol, smoking, obesity, diabetes, and physical inactivity. It has also yielded a great deal of valuable information on the effects of related factors such as blood triglyceride and HDL cholesterol levels, age, gender, and psychosocial issues. Although the study participants are primarily white Americans, the importance of the major risk factors identified in this group have been shown in other studies to apply almost

universally among racial and ethnic groups, even though the patterns of distribution may vary from group to group.

4. A third generation (the children of the Offspring Cohort) is currently being recruited and examined, seeking to further understand how genetic factors relate to cardiovascular disease.

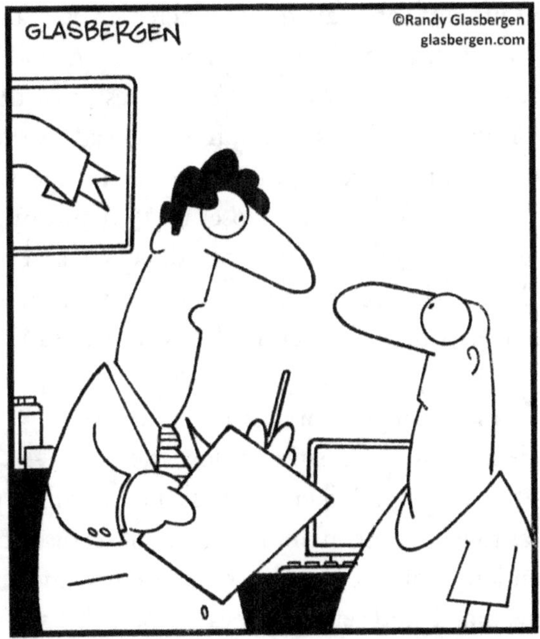

"The good news is, you have the heart of a teenager. The bad news is, most teenagers these days have the heart of an old man."

Risk factors can be divided into two broad categories: modifiable, or ones you can control, and non-modifiable, which you cannot control.

Let's start with the non-modifiable ones first.

Age and sex

Samarth Bansode was 25 years old and had just completed his job interview for a banking position in the beginning of March 2012 and was awaiting the outcome. On the morning of the 25th, he awoke feeling nauseous, and threw up. After a while he went back to sleep but was awakened with a dull pain in his left arm. He was taken to a hospital, where he was diagnosed with a heart attack. Samarth was in the ICU recovering from his heart attack when he got the call from the bank, saying that he'd got the job. At this point, he was in no position to accept the job, and heart disease had claimed one more victim.

Much as we may hate to admit it, age is a one-way street. In simple words, as we grow older, our risk for heart disease increases. Research has shown that if you are a man older than 45, or a woman older than 55, your risk for heart disease increases. This is based on Western research, though there is data to show that Indians tend to suffer almost a decade earlier. While this is not a published guideline, in my opinion, the cut-off age for Indian men should be closer to 35 and for women, closer to 45. Unfortunately, you are never too young to suffer (as we saw in Samarth's case), and what was once considered an 'old man's disease' is now routinely seen in those below 40. It is fairly common to see patients in their mid-30s, and at least once a month, I see someone below the age of 30.

On the other hand, though heart disease is the leading cause of death in women, it's rare to see women suffer below the age of 40. So, why this reverse discrimination for men? Whenever I ask a room full of patients (who are mostly men), as to why more men suffer from heart disease, I get a lot of grins, and the standard reply is, 'Women give us stress and therefore heart disease.' While a woman could certainly break a man's heart, that's not quite the same as giving him heart disease. The true reason is to do with hormones. The female hormone oestrogen is thought to provide protection against heart disease, which is why women suffer more after menopause. In that sense, after menopause, heart disease is an equal opportunity killer and is the leading cause of death worldwide in both men and women. In the recent past, some studies have emerged which suggest that menopause does not really increase a woman's risk, and that the increased risk is just a function of aging. More research needs to be done to see if that's indeed true.

Family history

Something else we cannot change is our family. I remember meeting with Mrs Sabina Gupta after her bypass surgery. As part of her medical history, I asked if anyone in her family had had heart disease, and her one word answer was, 'Everyone.' Naturally, I thought she was exaggerating a little bit, and asked her to give me more details. She then went on to describe her family's extensive history of heart disease. After an hour's discussion, I discovered that all six of her mother's brothers had heart disease, with three of them suffering before the age of 50. Her mother also had two sisters, both of whom suffered heart disease. As if that was not bad enough, her father and all three of his brothers had heart disease, along with all three of his sisters. Clearly, Sabina had the odds hugely stacked up against her, and ultimately needed to have bypass surgery at the age of 53.

There is a genetic risk associated with heart disease, which is highest if your parents or siblings have suffered. However, by no means is it a fait accompli— it just means that your risk is higher as compared to someone whose parents did not have heart disease. Sometimes, if the genetic lottery has handed you a ticket like Sabina's, then it may be very difficult to completely avoid heart disease. However, early vigilance and care might make the difference between dropping dead at 50 versus living with controlled heart disease till 85.

As our understanding of genetics increases, scientists are constantly on the hunt for variations in gene structure which might identify those at higher risk for heart disease. These variations are known as single-nucleotide polymorphisms (SNP—pronounced as 'snip'). There are about 30 sites in the DNA sequence which have been identified as increasing the risk of a heart attack when there is a variant presence. I am currently involved in a study looking at the presence of SNPs in an Indian population. At present, genetic testing is not yet used in clinical practice since we have not fully understood the clinical relevance of these SNPs. However, the day is not far when we will be able to identify those at risk through genetic testing, and be able to tailor treatment based on these results, a concept known as 'personalized medicine'.

Risk factors that we can change

Smoking and tobacco use

Smoking is among the largest causes of preventable death in the world. It's the leading risk factor for heart disease, stroke, lung and uterine cancer. The toxins in cigarette smoke damage the inner lining of the coronary arteries, which often initiates the process of atherosclerosis. Besides this direct effect, smoking decreases the HDL or good cholesterol in the body. In addition, smoking tends to cause spasm of the heart arteries. Quitting smoking is one of the hardest lifestyle changes to achieve, but it's also the most rewarding. The good news is that, after quitting, a smoker's risk drops rapidly, and in five years, the risk is almost that of a non-smoker. Besides smoking, tobacco is also consumed in the smokeless form. Many users quit smoking and take up tobacco use in the mistaken belief that they are doing less harm to themselves. Going by the many dangers of tobacco use, this is like jumping from the frying pan into the fire.

The Global Adult Tobacco Survey India (2009–2010) revealed that more than one-third (35 per cent) of adults in India use tobacco in some form or the other. This is a shocking number and translates into 275 million Indians consuming tobacco in some form. In fact, so addicted are we to this plant that we use it in every possible way, including smoking, chewing, applying, sucking, gargling, and inhaling it as snuff. We are the third-largest producer and second-largest consumer of tobacco worldwide.

In all areas of heart-healthy living we preach the path of moderation, but this is one area where moderation is not good enough. If you currently smoke, then you need to make a serious effort to quit. Often, on being asked about smoking, patients say that they have a cigarette occasionally. Now in my mind, the word occasionally translates to once in a week or so. However, after questioning thousands of patients, I realize that everyone uses the word differently to suit their convenience, and more than once I have learnt that the patient's version of 'occasionally' translated to once a day. Most smokers accept that they have a problem, but are so addicted to the habit that, when I counsel them to quit, they will try and rationalize with me (and themselves) how a cigarette once in a while won't hurt them. They also try to convince me that since they were smoking 15 cigarettes a day earlier, wouldn't it be okay if they cut it down to five cigarettes a day. My answer to them is a well-rehearsed one, since I have said it a hundred times. I tell them, it's like asking me whether it's better to jump off the fifteenth floor of a building, or jump off the fifth floor! They usually get the message.

High blood pressure or hypertension

Blood pressure (BP) is the force exerted by your blood on the walls of your arteries as it moves through the body. It is expressed in millimetres of mercury (mmHg), and consists of two numbers. The upper number, called systolic BP, is the force exerted when the heart is contracting (systole), while the lower number is during the relaxation phase of the heart cycle, and is called diastolic BP. A large percentage of the population has high blood pressure and does not know about it, since there are no specific symptoms of high BP. Most people have the wrong notion that if their BP is high they will get headaches, but the fact is that most people with high BP do not get headaches, and most headaches are not caused by high BP. This is the reason why high BP is known as the silent killer.

Another problem when it comes to detecting and treating high BP is the confusion over what's a normal number. Decades ago, doctors used to believe that your upper number should be 100 plus your age, so if you were 50 years old, it would be 'normal' to have a systolic BP of 150. Today, 150 is considered a very high number and normal BP is less than 120/80. (See table on the next page for complete classification of BP.) A common question asked is, below which number is BP considered too low. There is no official cut-off for low BP, also called hypotension. As a general guideline, if your BP is below 100/70, you should make your doctor aware of it. Your blood pressure is considered low if you have symptoms such as fatigue, dizziness and fainting. It is quite common for young women to have their pressure in the range of 90/60, who feel fine, and they should not be labelled as hypotensive.

There is another myth that your lower number (diastolic BP) is more important and that's what matters, irrespective of your systolic BP. Research has shown that both numbers are equally important. In fact, starting from a BP of 110/70, your risk for cardiovascular disease (heart attack and stroke) doubles with every 20 points increase in your systolic blood pressure, and 10 points increase in your diastolic blood pressure.

Category	Systolic BP (mmHg)		Diastolic BP (mmHg)
Normal	< 120	And	< 80
Pre-hypertension	120-139	Or	80-89
Hypertension, stage I	140-159	Or	90-99
Hypertension, stage II	>160	Or	> 100

Cholesterol

It was in the mid-1960s that researchers discovered the link between high cholesterol and heart disease, but it wasn't until the mid-1980s that cholesterol received much public attention. In 1984, an iconic *Time* magazine cover had two fried eggs and a sausage placed on a plate to represent a sad face, with the headline: 'Cholesterol: And now the bad news…'. The cover story went on to say, 'Cholesterol is proved deadly, and our diet may never be the same. This year began with the announcement by the Federal Government of the results of the broadest and most expensive research project in medical history. Its subject was cholesterol, the vital yet dangerous yellowish substance whose level in the bloodstream is directly affected by the richness of the diet. Anybody who takes the results seriously may never be able to look at an egg or a steak the same way again.'

Blood pressure is considered the silent killer, but if anything, cholesterol is even more silent. Cholesterol is a waxy substance, which is an essential component forming the walls of our cells. It also helps in the formation of some of the hormones in the body. While cholesterol is essential for normal living, when present in excess, it gets deposited in the lining of the coronary arteries and starts the process of plaque formation.

The major portion of our cholesterol is made in the liver, but it is also consumed in the food we eat. Only foods of animal origin contain cholesterol, including milk. In fact, milk and milk products are a major source of dietary cholesterol in the Indian vegetarian diet. In addition, the saturated fat that we consume in our diet is also converted to cholesterol in the body. Saturated fat tends to raise blood cholesterol levels more than the direct cholesterol we eat, and is present in both vegetarian and non-vegetarian food. This explains

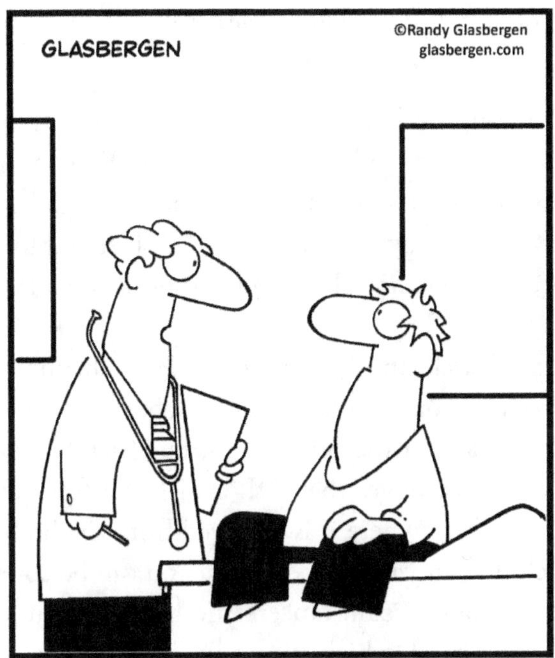

"Yes, garlic and herbs can improve your cholesterol...but not garlic and herb potato chips."

why vegetarians are not immune to high cholesterol levels. This also explains why in 1999, the *Time* magazine cover had two fried eggs and a slice of melon placed on a plate to represent a happy face, with the headline: 'Cholesterol: And now the good news…'. The egg had lost its evil status and once more become an acceptable part of our diet. This is because both eggs and shell fish (such as prawns) contain a high level of cholesterol, but are remarkably low in saturated fat, and can be consumed in controlled portions as part of a healthy diet.

Cholesterol is transported in the body in the form of lipoproteins (combination of fat and protein). The different components of your cholesterol profile, also called lipid profile, include:

1. Total cholesterol
2. LDL (low density lipoprotein) cholesterol

3. HDL (high density lipoprotein) cholesterol
4. Triglycerides

People often come up and say, 'Doctor, we can never remember which one is the good cholesterol and which one is bad.' Early on in my career, I learned from my mentor, Dr Neil Gordon (one of the global leaders in the field of preventive cardiology), to remember that 'L' stands for lousy, so LDL cholesterol is the bad one, and 'H' stands for healthy, so HDL cholesterol is the good one.

LDL cholesterol sticks inside your arteries, and the more the LDL in a plaque, the softer it becomes and greater the chances of it rupturing, and causing a heart attack. On the other hand, our friend, HDL cholesterol, goes and removes or scavenges the LDL cholesterol from the arteries and takes it to the liver, from where it is removed from the body. Triglycerides are the fats which flow in your blood stream and can be converted to LDL cholesterol under certain circumstances. Another term you may have come across is VLDL cholesterol, which is actually a component of triglycerides, and you need not worry about it separately.

From all the lipid profile components, LDL cholesterol is considered the most dangerous, and is the primary target of therapy. The question which has confronted cardiologists is, how low should you go? Current guidelines state that those with heart disease and diabetes should have their LDL below 100 mg/dl, and if it can be brought down to below 70 mg/dl, that would be even better. In private conversations I have had with some of the best cardiologists in the world, they suggest that 50 mg/dl may be the perfect LDL level to target.

Goal values for your lipid profile

Total cholesterol :	Less than 200 mg/dl
Triglycerides :	Less than 150 mg/dl
LDL cholesterol :	Less than 100 mg/dl (less than 70 mg/dl would be even better)
HDL cholesterol :	More than 40 mg/dl

Your cholesterol values should not be interpreted in isolation, but should take into account the presence or absence of other risk factors. Most people with high cholesterol are reluctant to get on medication, and will go to great lengths to avoid it. They are keen on solving the problem through lifestyle changes. In my opinion, there are three factors which go into determining your lipid profile: your diet, your physical activity pattern, and genetics. For simplicity sake, let's assume that each of them plays an equally important role. When a patient has high cholesterol, my decision to initiate medication will depend upon the overall risk profile, as well as the current lifestyle led by the person. Let's look at an example of two different persons with bad readings on their lipid profile. The irony is that I would be more likely to start medication for the one currently leading a good lifestyle, and will hold off on medication for the person leading a 'bad' lifestyle. Let me explain this seemingly bizarre logic. If someone is already exercising appropriately and eating a healthy diet, then there isn't much scope for improvement, and hence he/she will need medication to improve the lipids. On the other hand, if they are doing everything wrong at the moment, from a lifestyle perspective, there is large room for improvement. They should be given a three-month trial to improve their numbers through diet and exercise before starting medication.

Diabetes

India has the dubious distinction of being the diabetes capital of the world. The presence of diabetes and the factors clustered around it are thought to be the cause of the high predisposition that Indians have towards heart disease. The damage done by diabetes to your blood vessels is so significant that if you have diabetes today, it's considered equivalent to having heart disease, and the care and guidelines are similar.

Diabetes is a disease of high blood sugar. Food that we eat is broken down to a simple sugar known as glucose, which is digested with the help of the hormone insulin. Diabetes occurs when the body does not make adequate insulin, or there is a resistance to the action of insulin. When your body does not make insulin, it is known as Type 1 diabetes, and is usually detected in childhood (earlier it was also known as juvenile diabetes). In Type 2 diabetes, there is usually an adequate amount of insulin, but the body is unable to use it appropriately, known as insulin resistance.

Diabetes acts by attacking the small and large blood vessels in different parts of the body, causing micro and macrovascular disease. Besides the arteries of the heart, diabetes commonly affects blood vessels in the kidney and the eyes, and also leads to loss of sensation in different body parts, especially your feet, by attacking the nerves.

Diagnosis of diabetes

Diabetes is diagnosed on the basis of your blood sugar (glucose) levels. Normal fasting sugar should be between 70–100 mg/dl, and post-meal level should be below 140 mg/dl. These are international guidelines, but sadly many of our labs still publish older values of normal, which only end up confusing patients. If your fasting level is between 100–125 mg/dl, it's termed 'pre-diabetes'. If it crosses 126 mg/dl, and/or your post-meal value is more than 200 mg/dl, you are diagnosed to have diabetes. Since blood sugar tends to fluctuate a little on a daily basis, two readings on separate occasions should be taken to confirm a diagnosis of diabetes.

Another test for diabetes, which is getting increasingly popular is haemoglobin A1-C, commonly referred to as HbA1C. It is also known as glycosylated haemoglobin. This test measures the average blood sugar over a three month period, and you are diagnosed as diabetic if your value is above 6.5 per cent.

Bear in mind that all of these values are for diagnosing diabetes. Once you have diabetes, fasting and post-meal values will differ with each individual and your personal physician should set the boundaries of your ideal numbers.

	Normal	Pre-diabetes	Diabetes
Fasting blood sugar	70 – 100 mg/dl	100 – 125 mg/dl	≥126 mg/dl
Post-meal blood sugar	< 140 mg/dl	140 – 199 mg/dl	≥ 200 mg/dl
HbA1C	< 5.7 per cent	5.7 – 6.4 per cent	≥ 6.5 per cent

Syndrome X

Joe Menezes was 49 years old when he first got his routine health check-up done. He was a manager in a pharma company, and led a sedentary life. His blood pressure was 140/88 mmHg; his HDL cholesterol was 34 mg/dl; his fasting sugar was 110 mg/dl and he was about 5 kilos overweight. His waistline had expanded since his wedding 20 years ago, and the 30-inch waist he was proud of had blossomed to 38 inches. If you look at the normal values for each of these risk factors, you would comment that his numbers were higher than normal, but not by much. In fact, in many ways you could call him the average Joe on the street. However, when he consulted with me, I told him that he had 'Syndrome X', which left him wondering what I was talking about.

Syndrome X sounds like the latest Hollywood sci-fi movie, but in reality it's a cluster of factors, which when present, predisposes you to heart disease. It is also called the 'metabolic syndrome', or 'insulin resistance syndrome', and is defined by the presence of at least three of the following five factors:

Risk Factor	Cut-off level
Waist circumference: men	> 35 inches*
Waist circumference: women	> 31 inches*
Triglycerides	> 150 mg/dl
HDL Cholesterol	
Men:	< 40 mg/dl
Women:	< 50 mg/dl
Blood pressure	> 130/85 mmHg
Fasting blood sugar	> 100 mg/dl

(*These are the waist circumference cut-offs for Indians—they are slightly lower than the cut-offs for Westerners.)

Several studies have found that close to 40 per cent of so-called healthy people have Syndrome X. Often, none of the individual numbers are really high enough for concern, and therein lies the danger—the danger of taking it casually. Those with Syndrome X have a higher tendency to develop diabetes, as well as heart disease.

Physical inactivity

People love to talk about how stressful the times we live in are, and how our forefathers did not have any of these modern-day diseases that afflict us. While they are partly true, they invariably forget to talk about an integral component of our forefathers' lives, which is physical activity. I am fortunate to live in a gated community, with its own private roads and gardens, and I routinely see young men getting on their scooters to travel a few metres. On the other hand, when I observe my 11-year-old daughter, I notice that she rarely walks; even in the house she is always running from room to room. What's more interesting is that when my nieces (one of whom is eight, and the other is six) come over, they are more active than my daughter in reverse order of age. We were born to be physically active creatures, and somewhere down the line, a false sense of prosperity has led us to abandon our natural instincts and depend on mechanized transport for the smallest of tasks. This is also the greatest reason for the extra kilos we have put on over the years, and have conveniently blamed it on metabolism, age and a hundred other reasons, except our own laziness.

Research has shown that regular physical activity can reduce the risk of heart disease by as much as 50 per cent. Besides heart disease, it can also reduce the risk for several other chronic diseases, such as stroke and cancer. On the other hand, new research is emerging which shows the ill effects of sedentary behaviour. There is growing evidence that inactivity is harmful for your body, irrespective of whether you exercise or not. In other words, it does not matter if you are someone who never exercises, or are a marathoner—the more time you spend sitting, the worse it is for your health.

Recently, I visited the Cleveland Clinic, which has been rated as the best cardiac hospital in the United States for the last 19 years consecutively. Out there, I had the good fortune of meeting with Dr Mike Roizen, the Chief

Wellness Officer. It was one of the most interesting meetings I have ever had, since he was walking at his desk, while I was sitting. Walking at his desk? That sounds crazy, but it's true—he has a 'treadmill work station'. A desk is created at standing height around a treadmill, which allows the person to walk at a slow pace of 1.5–2 kilometres per hour while continuing to work. Dr Roizen is co-author of the best-selling book, *YOU: The Owner's Manual,* along with Dr Mehmet Oz (cardiac surgeon and host of the famous *Dr Oz Show*). He believes that one can defy aging with the correct health approach, and clearly practices what he preaches. In fact, companies such as Google and Microsoft now have treadmill work stations in some of their offices.

My good friend and colleague, Dr John Buckley, is the Chairman of the International Council of Cardiovascular Prevention and Rehabilitation. He is also a professor at the University of Chester, UK, where he has done research which shows that standing up for three extra hours per day would burn off around 4 kg of fat each year. Dr Buckley often uses a 'standing desk', which can be created by simply adjusting the height of your desk, and may be more practical than a treadmill desk.

While it may sound strange, this concept has been around for a long time. Great leaders such as Thomas Jefferson and Winston Churchill, and the writers Ernest Hemingway and Charles Dickens are reputed to have used standing desks. I would recommend that you try and take a standing break of at least a few minutes for every hour you spend sitting. Which reminds me—I need to take a break now and get off my seat.

Fitness does not provide immunity

Purshottam Ail was 15 years old when he won the prize for best all-round athlete at the Government High School in Mangalpady, Kerala, in 1960. On July 1, 2013 he won the gold medal in discus throw and silver in shot put at the National Masters Athletic Championship in Bangalore, at the age of 68. He was selected to represent India at the World Masters Athletic Championship to be held in October, in Brazil. Alas, that was not to be. Instead, on the 5th of August, he had to have an angioplasty for two blocked arteries.

Mr Ail and everyone around him were surprised that it had happened to him. Actually, shocked would be a better word. He was so fit, and had been since childhood. How did he land up with heart disease? This is a question which arises every time someone who exercises gets heart disease. I tell my patients that asking how a fit person could get heart disease is like asking how could you have an accident if your car's brakes are working perfectly. That the brakes are working well—though important—is just one aspect of 'not having an accident'. Similarly, just because you are fit does not mean you cannot have heart disease. As we have seen, there are several other risk factors that contribute towards having a problem.

When I went through Mr Ail's medical history in detail, I noticed that he'd had high BP for a few years, and his cholesterol was above the normal range. No doubt, fitness gives you protection against heart disease, but it does not give you immunity.

Obesity

This is the biggest (pun intended) problem that developed societies are facing today. Unfortunately, India is suffering from the twin burden of under-nutrition and low body weight in the poor segments of society, and over-nutrition in the economically prosperous segments. Stand at the entrance of any popular mall on a Sunday morning and watch the families leaving. A very large number of them, especially the children, are visibly overweight, and carrying the obligatory can of soft drink and packet of chips in their hands.

Obesity is today considered to be the fifth largest cause of preventable death in the world. However, in my personal opinion, it is made out to be a bigger villain than it is, and while that sounds controversial, here is my reasoning. Several scientific studies have shown that you can be overweight and healthy at the same time if you exercise regularly and eat the correct type of food. It can be argued that it's not the obesity per se, but the factors that get you obese which are responsible for the higher incidence of diseases associated with the condition. One may call that splitting hairs, since a large percentage of obese people have got there due to faulty lifestyles, but it also explains why there are so many obese people who do not suffer from heart disease. Conversely, there are many thin people who lead an unhealthy lifestyle and suffer from heart disease.

How do you define obesity?

Obesity is excess body fat. There are many different ways in which this can be assessed, and each has its pros and cons. The most common methods used to determine body fat are body mass index (BMI) and waist circumference.

• **Body mass index (BMI)**: This is an index of your weight in relation to your height and is the preferred method used by doctors at present.

How to calculate your BMI

- Step 1: Find out your weight in kilograms (kg)
- Step 2: Find out your height in cm (height in cm = height in inches x 2.54)
- Step 3: Convert your height to metre (cm/100)
- Step 4: BMI = weight in kg / (height in m)^2
- Eg. If your weight is 70 kg and your height is 5 ft 9 inches
- Height: 5'9' = 69 inches = 175 cm = 1.75 m
- BMI = $70/1.75^2$ = 22.9 kg/m^2

Your ideal BMI should be between 18.5 and 25. A BMI higher than 25 is considered overweight, and more than 30 is considered obese (see table below).

BMI Classification

	BMI (KG/M²)
Underweight	Less than 18.5
Normal	18.5-24.9
Overweight	25.0-29.9
Obesity, Grade I	30.0-34.9
Obesity, Grade II	35.0-39.9
Severe obesity	More than 40

These are the international criteria for BMI, but over the years research has shown that Asian men and women tend to suffer from diseases such as diabetes and hypertension at a much lower BMI than their Western counterparts. They discovered that for the same BMI values, Asians tend to store a lot more body fat than Westerners. In 2004, the World Health Organization (WHO) and several others since then have suggested a lower cut-off for Asian populations. They have not changed the official classification, but have suggested 23 kg/m^2 as a 'public health action point' for normal weight, and 27.5 kg/m^2, for obesity.

BMI is quick and easy to calculate, but the criticism is that it tends to overestimate body fat in those who are muscular, since it's not actually measuring fat, but using weight as a surrogate measure. Also, fat in the body is not evenly distributed and the location of fat is as important as the total amount present. Fat stored in the abdomen has shown to be metabolically more active, and leads to diabetes and heart disease. On the other hand, fat stored around the hips and thighs is actually found to be protective. You may have come across the descriptions 'apple-shaped' and 'pear-shaped'. An apple-shaped person is one in whom fat is stored around the stomach, which is dangerous, and is usually seen in men. On the other hand, pear-shaped fat is when the fat accumulates around the hips and thighs, more commonly seen in women. Women may despair at this accumulation of cellulite and spend hours trying to get rid of it, but the good news is that this fat may actually be beneficial (though women probably won't take solace in this).

• **Waist circumference:** In addition to BMI, another simple but excellent method of estimating body fat is by measuring the waist circumference. Men who have a waist circumference greater than 40 inches, and women with a waist more than 35 inches, are considered overweight. Again, there are different criteria for Asians, with 35 inches being the cut-off for men and 31 inches for women. The waist circumference should be measured at the narrowest part of your torso, between your navel and chest. Do not measure it at the navel, since that spot will shift, depending on weight gain or loss. In my opinion, a combination of BMI and waist circumference will give you an accurate picture of your risk. In addition, some of the other methods used to estimate body fat are:

• **Bio-electric impedance**: This is a method by which body fat is estimated by passing a small electric current through the body. Don't worry, you won't feel anything. It's extremely common in gyms, and now several home models are available too, but they are not very accurate. Often they are integrated as part of the weighing scale.

• **Skin fold callipers**: These callipers are used to measure skin fold thickness at various sites in the body. It is based on the assumption that the fat just below your skin (subcutaneous) is representative of your overall fat content.

• **DEXA scan**: Dual energy X-ray absorptiometry scans are primarily used to measure bone density, but can also be used to measure body fat in various segments. You need to lie down on an examination table, and a scanner moves over your body, measuring fat in different areas. This is probably the most accurate method of measuring body fat, but also the most expensive.

Easy BMI calculator

BMI – KG/M^2	21	23	25	27	30
YOUR HEIGHT (in feet and inches)	YOUR WEIGHT IN KG				
5.0'	49	53	58	62	69
5.1'	50	55	60	65	72
5.2'	52	57	62	66	74
5.3'	54	59	64	69	77
5.4'	56	61	67	72	80
5.5'	57	63	68	73	82
5.6'	59	65	71	76	85
5.7'	61	67	72	78	87
5.8'	62	68	74	80	89
5.9'	64	70	77	83	92
5.10'	67	73	79	86	95
5.11'	68	75	81	88	97
6.0'	70	77	84	91	101

Stress

In the course of my practice, I have come across many interesting patients, and Shailendra Kothari is one of them. He is a 54-year-old brand consultant who drives business development through corporate marketing and communication. Shailendra, known to his friends as Shailu, underwent bypass surgery recently. After taking his medical history, I was struck by the fact that he was truly one of those individuals whom I would label as unlucky from a medical point of view. He did not have any risk factors for heart disease and had led a disciplined life right from the start. He was genetically lucky too, since his father was 90 years old and in great health. I found his story interesting, and asked him to share it. I am reproducing it here, in his words. After all, he is an expert in communication.

That night it seemed like I had overeaten. Though I hardly ever do so! A feeling of indigestion. And it occurred again the next day, which sent me scurrying to my family doctor. The walk seemed to sort of exacerbate the feeling of indigestion. That day and the entire next week went by in a flurry. The immediate stress test that the doctor ordered led to more tests, and an angio that revealed more than I could ever conceive or wish to! And an eventual bypass surgery.

I have led a somewhat active life (well, in any case, not sedentary); been quite careful with my food habits (being a vegetarian besides). I do not smoke, consume alcohol or tobacco.

So what takes?

And this, compared to my father, who is 90 now, sedentary for the last couple of decades, eats (fried included), drinks and has made merry all through his life.

So what takes?

I think it's how he and I have approached life and living. He doesn't stress; I do. He isn't exacting; I am. He doesn't become overwrought; I do. He takes it easy; I don't. The vicissitudes of life he takes in his stride and on the chin; I don't. Everything for him is 'all right'; not for me.

That is what it takes! Not for cholesterol, or ABC or XYZ. Your demeanour to things, to persons around you, your mindset, your attitude. The living of life with grace, gratitude and giving.

In any public seminar, when I ask a group of people as to what they think is the main cause of heart disease, without fail, the answer is 'Stress'. Interestingly, stress was not considered one of the traditional risk factors, though there is growing evidence now that it is strongly linked with heart disease. A landmark study, known as The InterHeart Study, which was conducted across 52 countries, showed that 'psychosocial factors' were one of the nine most important causes for heart disease. Psychosocial factors include stress, anxiety and depression. It also includes, as we saw in Mr Kothari's case, your attitude to life. The reason why stress and associated factors become difficult to study is that they cannot be measured the same way as we can measure BP or cholesterol. Since we cannot measure it, it also becomes hard to define. Stress is a normal part of life, which when present in the right amount helps us function optimally, but when stress becomes excessive, it turns to distress. Often the same event can be a source of 'good' stress to someone, and a source of distress to another. I remember my good friend Dr Hetal Chiniwala (who is now a well known orthopaedic surgeon) used to throw up an hour before all our final MBBS exam papers. On the other hand, there were students who had a good night's sleep before the exam, and seemed least concerned (outwardly, at least). We all had the same stress (the exams), but all of us handled it differently. The interesting part of the story is that even though he was clearly stressed, he managed to be ahead of most of the class in every subject!

Stress is an 'independent' risk factor for heart disease, but it also acts via its influence on other risk factors such as high blood pressure, cholesterol and obesity. Due to stress, certain hormones are released which cause the heart to beat faster, and at the same time lead to a narrowing of the coronary arteries. A chronic state of stress may also cause the heart to develop abnormal rhythms, raise blood pressure, and even cause the release of cholesterol into the bloodstream.

Unhealthy eating

As I mentioned above, I've seen that—within the public seminars I address—most people perceive stress to be the leading cause of heart disease. The second-most common answer I get is 'bad eating habits'.

Food is essential for our survival and at the same time it contributes to most of the chronic health conditions that we suffer from. Just like exercise, the food we consume has an impact on cardiac risk factors, especially diabetes, cholesterol, blood pressure and obesity.

Aided by diet gurus, and the multi-billion dollar weight loss and nutrition industry, we tend to demonize some foods and elevate others to the status of super-foods. People get focused on individual food items and lose sight of the big picture. At the end of the day, the food that you consume over an extended period of time is what will determine your health outcome, and not individual meals. Your goal should be to follow a healthy diet over a lifetime, and not get too caught up with temporary fads. There is much debate on what constitutes a healthy diet, and I have devoted an entire section on nutrition to discuss in depth this important part of our daily lives. There will be enough information to digest at that point, which is why I haven't gone into detail at this juncture.

Newer risk factors

Rajnish Rathore was 37 years old and sitting in his office when he felt a sense of heaviness across his chest. At first he attributed it to acidity and ignored it, but when it persisted for several hours, he went across to the hospital, where it was diagnosed as a heart attack. Thanks to prompt medical attention, he survived the event, but could not come to terms with the fact that it had happened to him. A large percentage of my patients have this same feeling, and usually after going through their history, I am able to point out at least a few risk factors which could have led to their heart disease. So when Rajnish was sitting across my desk and asked, 'Why me?' I went through the list of usual suspects. I questioned him on his family history, blood pressure, cholesterol, smoking, obesity and diabetes, and realized that he had none of them. He seemed to truly belong to those unlucky few who had no obvious risk factors for heart disease but still suffered.

I then suggested that he measure his C-reactive protein, homocysteine and lipoprotein (a) levels, and they turned out to be high. It's due to cases like Mr Rathore that doctors are constantly on the search for 'newer' risk factors for heart disease, which might explain why some people who don't have the conventional risk factors still suffer. Over the last couple of decades, there have been several such discovered, chief among them being lipoprotein (a), highly sensitive C-reactive protein (hs-CRP), and homocysteine.

Lipoprotein (a), which is called 'L.P. little A', is a type of cholesterol particle which causes an increase in the 'stickiness' of blood cells, promoting clot formation, leading to a heart attack. Doctors are still not sure of the best way to tackle this risk factor, since it's not affected much by diet and exercise. One of the only medications to reduce it is niacin, but it's not known whether reducing Lp (a) through niacin can lead to reduced disease and increased longevity.

Another cholesterol-related test which is not done routinely is LDL particle size. We know that LDL is the bad cholesterol, but recent research has shown that, within LDL, there are two types. Some LDL particles are small and dense and these are more dangerous, while the larger ones are less damaging to the arteries.

Homocysteine is an abnormal protein, which is a by-product of certain chemical reactions taking place in the body. The mechanism by which it leads to increased heart disease risk is not yet clearly understood. Studies have shown that Indians tend to have a higher level of homocysteine as compared to Westerners.

C-reactive protein (CRP) is a protein found in the blood, the level of which rises in response to inflammation in the body. Studies have found elevated levels of CRP in those with cardiovascular disease, and it's thought to be a risk factor for heart disease. However, there is still a debate on whether an elevated CRP is a cause of heart disease, or whether it's simply associated with heart disease, but not a cause. When checking for it in your blood, you need to test for the highly sensitive fraction of it, also known as hs-CRP.

These newer risk factors are not routinely measured in all patients with heart disease or those at risk. It has been found that once the traditional risk factors are measured and a risk profile is created, these newer factors do not add any further predictive value. However, we usually measure them in young people with heart disease and no obvious risk factors, as well as those who have a strong family history of heart disease at a young age as a preventive measure.

What's your overall risk?

Your overall risk will depend on the total number of risk factors you have, as well as the level of each one of them. Have a look at the risk factor table below, score yourself on each of the risk factors, and total your score at the end. Please note that this table has been formulated by me to give you a sense of your overall risk, and is based on my experience, not on a standardized risk assessment score.

RISK FACTOR	POINTS			
	0	1	2	COMMENTS
Family history of heart disease (parents or siblings)	No heart disease	One family member	Two or more family members	
Smoking/tobacco	Never smoked	Quit	Current	Quit – for at least 3 months
Blood pressure	Below 130/85	130-140/ 85-90	More than 140/90	Add 1 point if on BP meds
Total cholesterol	Below 200	200-240	Above 240	Add 1 point if on cholesterol meds
Fasting blood sugar	Below 100	100-125	More than 125	Add 1 point if on diabetes meds
Body mass index (BMI)	Below 25	25-30	Above 30	
Physical activity	150 min or more per week	60-150 min per week	Less than 60 min a week	

Interpretation

Add up the points. Remember to add one point extra to your BP, cholesterol and sugar score if you are taking medication for these conditions. If you do have established diabetes, then it is automatically considered as high risk for heart disease.

0: Perfect score. All your risk factors are under great control, and your risk for heart disease is very low. Keep it up.

1–2: Good. Your risk is on the lower side. Work a little harder for the perfect score.

3–6: Moderate risk. You need to work on lowering your risk. Do consult your doctor.

7–9: High risk. If you have not consulted a doctor, make sure you do so right away, to advise you further

10+: Very high risk. You have several risk factors, which are not under control. Consult your doctor and get further cardiac testing done.

One plus one is not two

It's those who have a cluster of several risk factors that are slightly out of control, who end up suffering years later, as compared to someone who may have just one risk factor way out of control. Borderline values tend to be dangerous because doctors and patients alike tend to take them lightly. On the other hand, very high values tend to be easier to deal with, since immediate action is taken. Risk factors for heart disease are multiplicative, which is why one plus one risk factor does not double your risk, it multiplies it. In the war against heart disease, there is no room for complacency. You need to strive towards keeping your numbers under aggressive control to avoid the signs and symptoms of heart disease, which we will talk about in the next chapter.

Take-home messages

- Heart disease is caused by the presence of risk factors, most of which can be controlled. It's like driving a car—the more careful you are in controlling your risk factors, the less the chance of an accident.

- Age, sex, and family history of heart disease are important risk factors which cannot be changed.

- Smoking is probably the most dangerous risk factor for heart disease. If you do smoke, you need to quit completely.

- High blood pressure, high cholesterol and diabetes are major risk factors and need to be kept under aggressive control.

- Obesity, physical inactivity, stress and poor eating habits are lifestyle factors which need to be monitored.

- Newer risk factors are constantly being discovered, such as C-reactive protein, homocysteine, and lipoprotein (a). It is debated whether they cause heart disease or are merely associated with it.

5

Symptoms of Heart Attack and Emergency Treatment

(Warning signs from the heart)

THE MONTH OF JANUARY 2008 WAS A TERRIBLE ONE FOR STOCK INVESTORS in India. The sub-prime mortgage crisis in the US had created turmoil in world markets, and though India was relatively insulated from it, the third week of January was a bloodbath on Dalal Street. On Monday the 21st, the Sensex crashed by 1,408 points, which was followed by a 2,000 points intra-day loss on Tuesday. The Sensex closed on Tuesday, with a loss of 875 points, and Hemant Parekh was an extremely stressed sub-broker when he got home late that night. He had personally not lost money, but many of his clients had, especially the 'satta players'. Over dinner, he barely made conversation with his wife Sushila, but kept rubbing his hand over his chest, and was in an irritable mood. He was experiencing heaviness in the chest region, above the stomach, which he attributed to acidity and gulped down a few spoonfuls of Gelusil.

After watching an hour of CNBC, it seemed to get worse and he began pacing up and down in the living room. Sushila suggested calling their family doctor, and the idea was immediately vetoed by Hemant, saying it was ridiculous to disturb him at this time of night. He took some Eno salts and let out a series of burps, and looked at Sushila in a meaningful manner, as if the sounds confirmed his diagnosis of acidity. An hour later, he was tossing in bed, unable to sleep, and he started sweating, even though the room was air-conditioned. After further debate the family doctor was finally called, and when he arrived 30 minutes later, he asked Hemant to be moved to the nearest hospital. After further protests, he was finally convinced, and they drove to the hospital in a cab. He collapsed as they reached the entrance and was proclaimed dead on arrival. Heart disease and the stock market had claimed another victim.

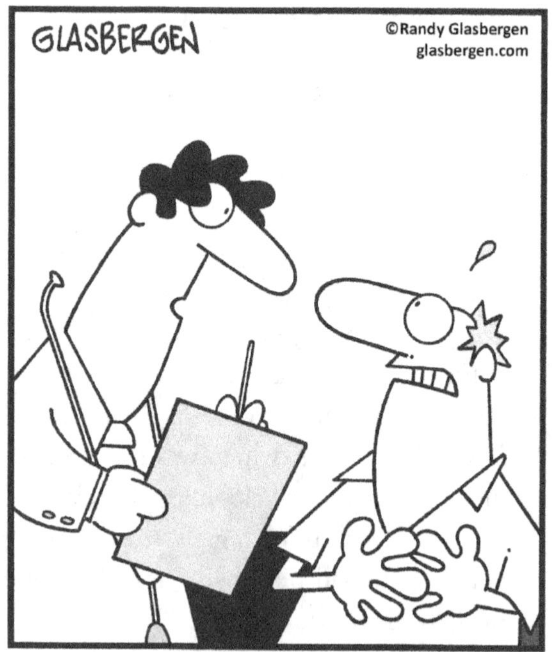

"It's normal for a man your age to have chest pains when he drips hot, melted pizza cheese on his shirt."

Heart attack symptoms may not be typical

In February 2012, Suresh Shinde had just returned from his native village Malvan, in the Konkan region of Maharashtra, after a four-day holiday. This region is famous for its coastal Malvani cuisine, and Suresh had made sure he did full justice to it during his vacation. The day he returned home to Palghar, on the outskirts of Mumbai, was Sankashti. Being a devout follower of Lord Ganesh, he fasted on that day. The next morning he woke up with a mild discomfort in the shoulder and back region, which he thought was muscle pain. He decided to hit the gym to make up for his feasting. After 45 minutes of exercise, the discomfort increased, and now he described it as a dull pain between the shoulder blades. To counter it, he took some painkillers, and when that did not help, he decided to go to a nearby clinic. At the clinic, an ECG revealed that he was having a heart attack and he was rushed to the nearest hospital, where he received thrombolysis treatment to dissolve the clot.

Suresh was diagnosed to have a massive anterior wall myocardial infarction (in simple words, the blood supply to a large part of the heart muscle on the front surface of the heart had been shut off, causing death of the heart muscle—a heart attack). A subsequent 2-D echo showed that his pumping capacity had been reduced to 25 per cent (from a normal of 55 per cent plus). He was lucky to have survived but permanent damage had been done. You may have heard the phrase, 'the golden hour', or another, 'time is muscle'. Both of these suggest that in a heart attack (or brain attack, known as stroke), the faster you get treatment, the higher the chances of survival without permanent damage. In Suresh's case, he had warning signs from 7 a.m. onwards, and received medical treatment only around 3 p.m., more than eight hours later. If he had received immediate help, it is possible that his heart muscle damage would not be quite as extensive, and his pumping capacity, or EF, would have remained normal. He was 29 years old at the time of the attack.

How do you know the pain is cardiac?

This is a tricky question since there are a number of different conditions which could give rise to discomfort in the chest region. Acidity and gas are the commonest, followed by muscle pain. As we saw in the examples above, Hemant mistook his pain for acidity, while Suresh mistook it for muscular pain. In both cases, it proved costly. Before we look at how to differentiate the conditions, it's worth looking at what is angina and how it manifests.

Angina pectoris is a Latin term meaning 'squeezing or strangling of the chest'. It occurs because a portion of the heart muscle is not receiving adequate blood supply, most likely due to a blockage in one or more of the coronary arteries. I have heard doctors describe it as 'the heart crying for blood'. Classic angina presents itself as pain in the left side of the chest, often radiating down to the left arm. However, more often than not, it does not present in this manner, and pain may occur anywhere in the chest region (left or right) and may radiate to either arm, or even the shoulders, back, and the jaw. To keep it simple, I tell my patients that anginal pain may occur anywhere from navel to nose. Also, the pain may manifest in different ways. Early on in my career, when I asked my patients about pain in the chest, they usually denied having any. After much probing and questioning they would say they had 'a heaviness in the chest'; some would call it 'burning'; but they rarely used the word 'pain'. Over time, experience has taught me to use the word 'discomfort' instead of 'pain', since that encompasses all uncomfortable sensations, whether it's pulling or tightness or any other descriptive term.

Angina is usually related to exertion, that is, the discomfort increases with activity and decreases with rest, while acidity or gas pain does not change much. Gas pain is more related with meals, though it is possible for angina to be present post meals too. My advice to patients is, when in doubt, assume it's angina and go to the nearest hospital right away. You should inform your family doctor, but don't wait for him or her to arrive, since time is crucial. If it is gas, worst case you will have lost some time, and a few hundred rupees, but if it is a heart attack you could be saving your life.

Other causes of chest discomfort

Pain in the chest region could also be related to respiratory causes, as well as stress and anxiety. Besides these, there are a number of cardiac causes of chest pain which are non-coronary. In other words, they are due to other types of heart diseases, and not atherosclerosis or blockage related and, frankly, it can be quite confusing to differentiate all of these. The most common causes of chest pain, however, are cardiac, gas related, and muscular.

I have made a simplified table to help you distinguish between cardiac, gas related, and muscular pains. However, I must stress that this is an extremely generalized approach, and huge individual variations in presentation do occur.

There are many patients in whom cardiac pain will present as gastric, and vice-versa. Therefore, if you do experience chest discomfort, seek medical help immediately.

Pain/Discomfort	Angina	Gastric- related	Muscular
Location of pain	Anywhere from navel to nose	Usually stomach area, below rib cage	Could be anywhere
Nature of pain	Dull, aching, constricting, burning. Rarely a sharp pain	Burning, aching. Could be sharp	Could be dull, or tender to touch
Spread of pain	Usually over a region, not at a specific point	Usually in a specific area	Usually in a specific area
Pain aggravated by	Physical activity	Usually after meals; not by physical activity	Muscular movement, or physical pressure at the site
Pain relieved by	Rest; Sorbitrate	Belching; antacids	Rest; painkillers

The difference between angina and heart attack

Before we discuss emergency steps, it's important to distinguish between angina and heart attack. Angina is pain related to the temporary reduction of blood supply to your heart muscle. It can come and go depending on your activity level. On the other hand, a heart attack is actual death of part of your heart muscle, also known as a myocardial infarction, or MI. If you are having a heart attack, the discomfort you will experience will be of a much higher intensity, as compared to angina. Many patients have described the pain of a heart attack as if an elephant is sitting on their chest. This pain is often accompanied by sweating, nausea, and sometimes a feeling of doom (like the whole world is collapsing on you). Several of my patients have complained of a sudden passing of stools (sometimes uncontrolled) during their heart attack. This is a sign which you don't read about in medical textbooks, but I have heard this often enough from my patients.

Is a cardiac arrest the same as a heart attack?

No. A cardiac arrest occurs when the heart suddenly stops functioning. It is caused due to a serious disturbance in the heart's electrical system. Often a heart attack leads to a cardiac arrest, but this is not always the case. A person in cardiac arrest will not be conscious and needs emergency treatment within a few minutes, or will not survive. Cardiopulmonary resuscitation, popularly known as CPR, should be initiated immediately. In addition, if there is a defibrillator available, it should be used to 'shock' the victim. You must have seen televisions serials such as *ER,* which are set in hospital emergency rooms, in which the doctors apply pads to a patient's chest and send a shock wave through the body. The machine that delivers the shock is called a defibrillator. The aim of this shock is to 'reset' the electrical system of the person's heart, with the hope that it will start functioning correctly after the reset. However, this may not always happen, and sometimes the person may remain in cardiac arrest. These days at airports, you often see glass cases with a small bag inside them, marked AED (Automated External Defibrillator). These are the 'shocking devices', which can be used by laypersons as well.

What is a silent heart attack?

This term is applied to heart attacks that are not accompanied by symptoms. Actually, let me rephrase that to heart attacks that do not have any symptoms or the symptoms are unrecognized.

Arshad Shaikh is a leading counsel in the Bombay High Court and a friend of mine from the gym. Arshad's father was my professor in biochemistry at T.N. Medical College as well as the warden of our hostel. Growing up in a medical environment, Arshad had a fair understanding of the subject, even though he took up law. Or maybe, that's why he took up law! So, when he came to meet me in my consulting room one afternoon, I was quite surprised. He told me that he had met with a doctor earlier in the day who had recommended an angiography for him. I went through his medical reports, and his ECG revealed that he'd had a heart attack in the past. He was taken aback with this news, since he was not aware of having any medical problems, leave alone a heart attack. On further probing, it turned out that about a month ago he'd had a prolonged episode of stomach bloating and breathlessness at night. He remained awake most of the night, sitting on his sofa. The next day he went to his family doctor, who gave him some antibiotics for the stomach. Over the next few days, he complained that he felt out of breath, but the family doctor attributed that to his use of antibiotics and no further tests were done. He felt uneasy for a few days, but then was back to normal. A few weeks later he went for a swim and felt fatigued after only half a lap and this alarmed him, since he was a seasoned swimmer. That is when he got an ECG done, and came to see me.

We got an angio done the next morning which revealed triple vessel disease. The results of the angio, coupled with the ongoing chest pain, prompted the cardiac team to take him up for an immediate bypass surgery.

In retrospect, the breathlessness and bloating he had a month ago was in all likelihood the symptoms of a heart attack, but since he did not consider it heart-related it was ignored, and hence labelled as a silent heart attack. Most people who have had a silent heart attack probably did get some symptoms, which they ignored. There are some, though, who do not get any symptoms at all. Those who have a silent attack are more prone to have another heart attack in the future, and need to be particularly watchful.

Women are more likely to have a silent attack than men. One of the reasons is that women, typically, do not get the classic pattern of angina and pain in the left side of the chest. They are more likely to present with atypical angina, in which they experience discomfort in the shoulders, back and neck. Often, shortness of breath is the first and only presenting symptom. This makes diagnosis difficult, since there are several causes of shortness of breath.

Diabetics are also more likely to have silent attacks. This is because diabetes also affects the nerves, which may lead to reduced sensations and therefore they may not experience the discomfort related to angina.

What should you do in case of an emergency?

A common question asked is whether any treatment measures can be begun at home in case of an emergency. Over the past few years, several e-mails have been circulating on the internet under the headline of, 'How to survive a heart attack when you are alone'. It suggests that you cough repeatedly and vigorously if you suspect you are having a heart attack. Unfortunately this is one of those e-mails which are circulated with good intention but not a good outcome, as this does not work.

- If you feel that you are actually experiencing a heart attack, you should first call for help. Have the number of a good ambulance service handy and get someone to call them. One-third of all heart attacks are fatal, and the faster you act the higher are your chances of survival.
- The best medical action you can take at that moment is to chew a tablet of aspirin. Usually aspirin is coated to prevent acidity, but in times of emergency you should use an uncoated aspirin so that it acts much quicker (Disprin is an example of uncoated aspirin). When taking aspirin in emergency, you should chew it first and then swallow it. The only time you should not take an aspirin is if you have an allergy to the tablet.
- I am often asked whether a Sorbitrate should be taken too. Sorbitrate is a well-known brand of medication, which is prescribed to relieve angina. If you have had heart disease in the past and have Sorbitrate (or similar medication) with you, then take one tablet and put it below your tongue. This helps it get absorbed much quicker into your system than swallowing it. Remember, when you take Sorbitrate, you need to be sitting or lying down because one of the effects of the drug is to lower your blood pressure. Therefore, if you take it in the standing position and your pressure drops precipitously, there is a chance of fainting and falling down. After you take the first tablet, wait for five minutes and see if you feel better. If you do not, then take one more tablet and wait for a further five minutes. If you do not get relief even after the second, then after five minutes take a third, and head to the nearest hospital for treatment.

Treatment for a heart attack

Before starting treatment at the hospital, the doctors will first confirm that it is indeed a heart attack. This is done by taking the patient's ECG and some blood tests. These tests measure the blood levels of enzymes which are typically found in your heart muscle. If you are having a heart attack, these are released into the bloodstream and are diagnostic.

In the setting of an acute heart attack, opening up the blockage is the best medical option. This is done by performing an angiography and then opening up the blockage with a balloon. This procedure is called an angioplasty and when done during the course of a heart attack, it's labelled PAMI—primary angioplasty in myocardial infarction. The time between onset of symptoms and angioplasty should be as little as possible, and should preferably be done within 12 hours (some studies suggest that it's okay up to 24 hours). The sooner it is done, the quicker the chances of a full recovery for the patient.

The other option for immediate treatment of a heart attack is thrombolysis. As the name suggests, this therapy causes 'lysis' or break down of a 'thrombus', which is the clot that plugs up the coronary artery during a heart attack. This is by far the most commonly used therapy in India due to reasons of availability and cost. Almost every hospital has the facility for thombolytic therapy, while very few have the ability to do a PAMI. For a successful PAMI program, the hospital needs to have a fully equipped cath lab (where angiography and angioplasty are performed), along with cardiologists and technicians on-call 24 hours of the day. In addition, there is a huge difference in cost, with thrombolysis costing approximately 25,000 rupees, and PAMI costing upwards of 2 lakh rupees. However, the outcomes are far superior with a PAMI, and it's what you should opt for if you or your loved ones are in the unfortunate position of needing one of these therapies. Angioplasty done while a person is having a heart attack is life-saving and a necessary procedure. However, when the person is stable, the decision-making is very different as is the need for the procedure. We shall discuss it further as we talk about the options for those with heart disease.

One important point I would like to repeat: when you are suspecting a heart attack, it is vital to get emergency help quickly. The sooner you get to a hospital the higher your chances of survival. In India it is customary to wait for the family doctor before making any decision. You should involve him or her, but make sure that does not delay your reaching the hospital. If your family doctor is not immediately available, let them meet you directly at the hospital, to save time and your heart.

Take-home messages

- Angina may present as any discomfort from navel to nose, which usually increases with exertion, and decreases with rest.

- It could be confused with gas or muscle pain. When in doubt, assume it's angina and get it checked.

- Symptoms of a heart attack are similar to angina, but in greater intensity. They are often accompanied with sweating, shortness of breath and a 'feeling of doom'.

- The best emergency care for a heart attack at home is to chew a tablet of aspirin and rush to the nearest hospital. Remember, a delay could mean further cardiac damage or death.

- At the hospital, the best emergency treatment is an immediate angioplasty (PAMI), and if that cannot be done, clot-busting drugs (thrombolysis) should be given.

6

Getting Diagnosed with Heart Disease: What Next?

(The next steps)

WHATEVER MAY BE YOUR VIEWS ON FORMER US PRESIDENT GEORGE W. Bush, there is no question that he is a very fit man. Throughout his presidency, from 2000–2008, he used to run and bike outdoors on a regular basis. He was known to be in very good health, so when he had an angioplasty done and a stent inserted in one of his arteries at a Texas hospital, it created big news. The procedure was done on August 6, 2013, and the same evening there were comments from cardiologists all across the US and the world on the lack of 'appropriateness' of the procedure. Just a week earlier, he had successfully completed a 100-km bike ride, and seemed to be in fine form. He then went in for a routine health check at the Cooper Clinic on August 5th, during which his stress test showed an abnormality. Almost immediately he underwent a CT angio, which showed a blockage, following which he was taken up for angioplasty. When this was announced, all hell broke loose within the cardiology community in the US, with strong words coming in from some very reputed cardiologists. Dr Steve Nissen, the head of Cardiology at the Cleveland Clinic said, 'This is really American medicine at its worst. It's one of the reasons we spend so much on healthcare and we don't get a lot for it. In this circumstance, the stent doesn't prolong life, it doesn't prevent heart attacks and it's hard to make a patient who has no symptoms feel better.' The Cleveland Clinic has been rated as the best cardiology centre in the US for the last 19 years consecutively, so clearly Dr Nissen's words carry great weight.

The reason for these reactions is that according to the latest 'appropriateness' guidelines issued by leading US cardiology associations, President Bush should not have undergone an angiography in the first place, and should certainly not have been stented.

Two large studies done over the past few years have shown that drug therapy works just as well as stents in preventing cardiac complications. These guidelines were therefore issued to avoid the rampant excessive stenting that was taking place in the US. To be fair to President Bush and his doctors, no one knows the full story, so it is possible that there were circumstances that we are not aware of which led to their decision. Was he a victim of what is known as the 'VIP syndrome', in which a person receives excessive treatment just because they are important?

This particular case got me thinking. Here was an apparently healthy person who seemed to be in the pink of health one day, and then, based on a test, was labelled as a heart disease patient and was intervened upon. Now he had to take certain medications for life, and go for follow-ups routinely.

Before we even talk about who should have an intervention, such as angioplasty and bypass surgery, it would be interesting to first look at what criteria we use to put the tag of 'heart disease patient' on someone.

When is a person said to have heart disease?

Mrs Mansukhani was a 68-year-old lady, whom I met for the first time during the course of a routine health check. She was accompanied by her husband. As part of the consult, my task was to determine her cardiac risk profile, and suggest ways to lower it. My first question to her was whether she had a history of heart disease, which she flatly denied. I then went on to review her lipid profile and other risk factors. As the end of the consult she folded her hands in a 'namaste', which is when I noticed a scar running on the inside of her arm. I asked her whether that scar was the result of a bypass surgery (surgeons often use the radial artery for the bypass graft), and she said yes. I reminded her that my first question was whether she had heart disease, to which she had replied in the negative. Her husband intervened and said that she did not have heart disease, but this was a 'preventive bypass surgery'. He explained that her stress test was positive a few years ago, and the angio showed some blockages. She was recommended a bypass surgery to prevent a heart attack, and that's what they did.

Mr Mansukhani's reaction is not unique. I have noticed that a large number of patients with heart disease (and their family members) do not acknowledge that they have it. I do not know whether it's denial or ignorance, but many think they have heart disease only if they have suffered a full-blown heart attack.

Nobody likes to be labelled as having heart disease, especially if they are young. The question that arises is, at what point does one apply this dreaded tag to an individual? Let's start with the easy end of the spectrum. If you have had a heart attack, confirmed by ECG and blood tests, then you clearly have heart disease. But what if you only had occasional chest discomfort on walking, which your doctor feels is 'nothing in all likelihood', but cannot rule out angina for sure? Or, what if you felt perfect, and on your routine annual check-up sponsored by your company, had a positive stress test, just like President Bush? In most of these cases, further testing is usually warranted and a combination of tests will help make a diagnosis.

It would be fair to say the diagnosis of heart disease is confirmed if you have any degree of blockages seen on your angiography or CT angio. It can also be confirmed based on results of your ECG, 2-D echo, or stress test, provided the results are clearly abnormal.

What to do after the angiography?

Mr Kirit Jain wore a confused look on his face when he came to consult me. I don't blame him, since he had just done a long round of visiting doctors for second and third opinions, and also had to contend with the opinions of his family members, four of whom had come along for the consult. He was a 55-year-old businessman who had recently had a mild heart attack, and a subsequent angiogram. The angio showed a blockage in his mid-LAD of 90 per cent, a blockage in his right coronary artery of 70 per cent and a non-significant block in his left circumflex artery. He had visited five cardiologists and surgeons, and had got different opinions from all. Two of them suggested surgery, two suggested angioplasty, and one said to do 'nothing at all' and continue medical management. To make it more confusing, one of the surgeons had suggested an angioplasty, and one of the cardiologists had suggested a bypass surgery. Even within the angioplasty team, there was a difference of opinion on how many stents needed to be used.

Many of you might identify with the plight of Mr Jain, since you or your family member might have faced the same dilemma. Patients go to doctors for second opinions to clear their doubts, but often they come back with more doubts. This practice of second and third and fourth opinions is known in the medical community as 'shopping around'. This usually happens when relatives and friends suggest different doctors and approaches that they always claim are the 'best' (I suppose they are doing it in good faith). Mr Jain wanted my suggestion on the way forward, which was a difficult call to take, given the circumstances.

Let me explain by starting at the beginning. Whenever a patient of mine has to undergo an angiography, they are always anxious to know the likely result and subsequent treatment. I tell them that there is a one-third chance they will not need an intervention and can be treated through medical management, or conservative treatment. There is a one-third chance that they may need angioplasty and one-third chance of a bypass surgery. I have found that this explanation helps them accept the final verdict when it does come, and they are not overly optimistic or pessimistic of the results.

To intervene or not, that is the question

After the angiography, the cardiologist and team of doctors need to make a decision on whether a patient needs a revascularization procedure, or to continue him or her on medical management. Revascularization means restoration of blood supply to the heart muscle. The choice of a revascularization procedure (also called interventional procedure) is between an angioplasty and bypass surgery. Ideally, this decision should be made by the 'heart team', and not just a single doctor. The team should consist of a cardiologist, cardiac surgeon, and the family physician, if available. Just to clarify, angiographies and angioplasties are done by cardiologists, while bypass surgery and other heart surgeries are done by a cardiac surgeon. I have often found that cardiac surgeons are called cardiologists, and patients are under the assumption that they do angiographies as well.

There are three main blood vessels which supply blood to the heart: the left anterior descending artery (LAD), the left circumflex artery (LCX) and the right coronary artery (RCA). You may have heard the term 'triple vessel disease', which refers to blockages in all three of these arteries. In earlier years the decision of when to do a bypass surgery and when to do an angioplasty was fairly clear-cut. If there was triple vessel disease, or left main artery blockage, you opted for surgery; if there was single vessel disease you opted for angioplasty; and with two vessel disease either choice was viable. In recent years the lines between surgery and plasty have blurred, with cardiologists often tackling left main disease as well as triple vessel disease through angioplasty.

In my personal opinion, which has been borne out through scientific studies, there are many situations in which multiple stents are inserted, when a bypass surgery would have been a better option. As a rule of thumb, if blockages are present in all three coronary arteries, then surgery is a better choice. In fact, even in most cases of double vessel disease, surgery is usually a better choice. Angioplasty is a good option in single vessel disease, and selected cases of double vessel disease. To be honest, the final decision is based on judgment and experience rather than exact science. There are several situations when all three options may be perfectly valid ones. In such situations, I prefer laying out the facts in front of the patient and family members, with the pros and cons of each option, and allow them to make their own decision. In our country, finance often plays a big role in the decision-making process, since most people do not have insurance or do not have enough insurance to cover the complete cost of the procedure. Worldwide, a bypass surgery is far more expensive than an angioplasty, but in our country, a bypass surgery is usually cheaper than an angioplasty, in situations where the angioplasty is followed by two or more stents.

With the number of possible cardiac tests, along with the various treatment options, as well as opinions of doctors and family and friends, it's quite possible that a cardiac patient may land up with a mental breakdown, rather than a heart attack! The flow chart on the following page will give you some idea on which might be the best procedure for you under different circumstances. However, do keep in mind that there are several factors which need to be taken into consideration when suggesting the right approach, and these differ from patient to patient. Your treating doctor will be in the best position to recommend the most appropriate treatment for you.

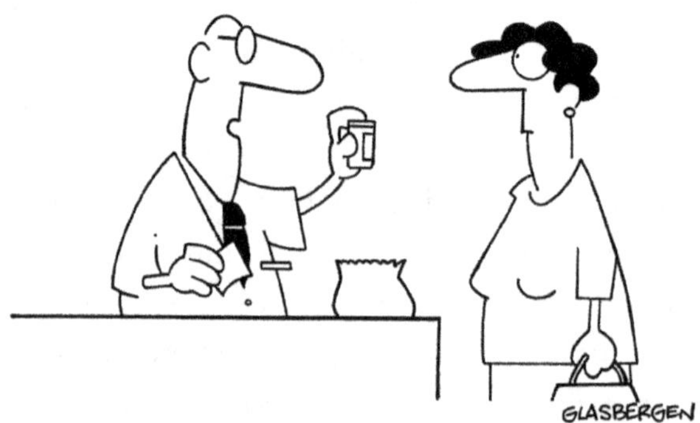

"This is one of those new miracle drugs.
If you can afford it, it's a miracle."

DECISION-MAKING FLOWCHART FOR PATIENTS WITH HEART DISEASE

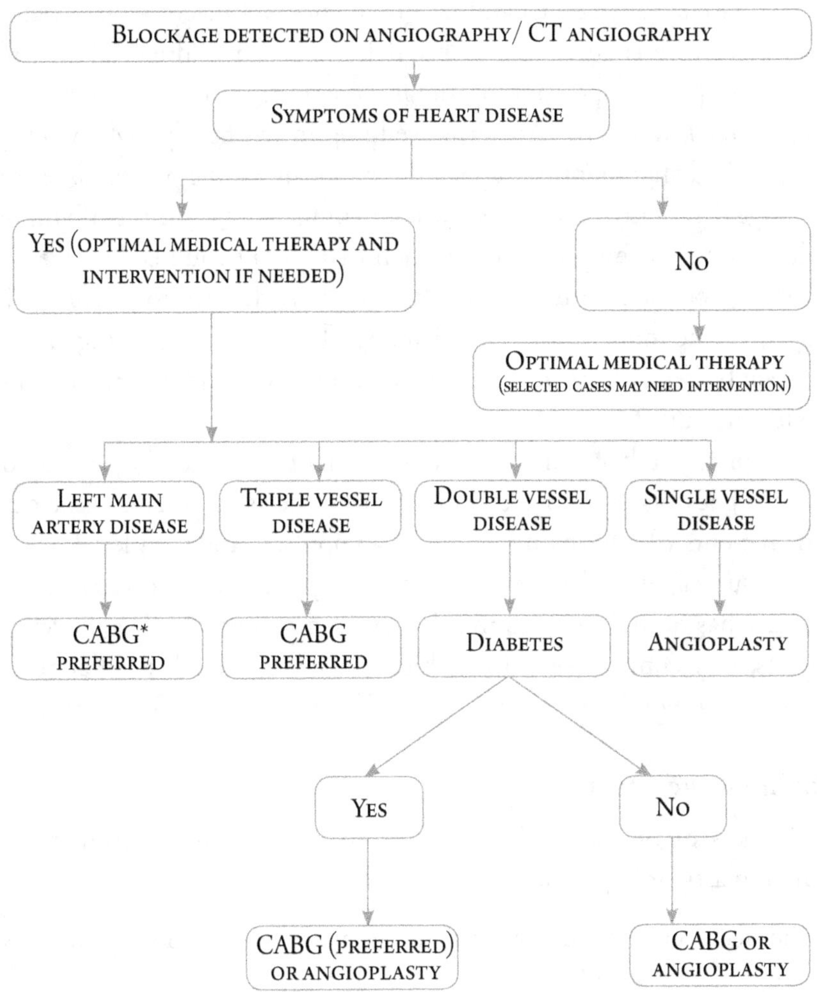

* CABG: CORONARY ARTERY BYPASS GRAFT SURGERY

Do it quickly

A word of advice to patients and family members. Once you have decided on a particular procedure, then do not delay in getting it done. All too often I have heard patients postponing the intervention for reasons such as, 'Let us do it after Diwali', or, 'After the wedding in the family'. Many delay it because of bad alignment of the planets, and wait for the perfect *muharat*. I discourage this in my patients, and the reasoning is very simple. If you have decided not to do anything further, then that's a call you need to live with, and timing does not matter. However, if you have decided to do something, then get it done sooner rather than later. God forbid, if something fatal was to happen because of the delay, family members will find it very difficult to live with the guilt.

Also, once you have undergone a particular procedure, there is no point in double-guessing if you have made the right decision. I have come across several patients who have undergone an angioplasty and wondered whether a bypass surgery would have been a better option and vice versa. Once a procedure has been done it cannot be reversed and the best way forward is to aggressively control your risk (which is what this book is all about), to make sure that you lead a great quality of life without any future problems.

Take-home messages

- All cases of blockages do not need to have an intervention such as angioplasty or bypass surgery.

- The decision on whether to intervene will depend upon symptoms as well as the results of your test.

- Appropriateness criteria have been laid down by international associations on which situations need aggressive medical management, angioplasty or bypass surgery.

7

Bypass Surgery

(Mending a broken heart)

THE MOST BIZARRE STORY I HAVE HEARD IN MY ENTIRE LIFE WAS TOLD TO me by one of my patients. Mr Abdul was a 65-year-old gentleman, who experienced severe chest discomfort on walking. His angiography showed triple vessel disease and he was recommended a bypass surgery. He wanted to avoid surgery at any cost and came to me in June 2003 for suggestions on alternate treatments.

When a patient has active angina and triple vessel disease, the best course of treatment is a bypass surgery, which is what I told him. He did not look too convinced, and I was quite sure I would never see him again. To my surprise, he turned up at my clinic two months later with a big smile on his face, and told me that his heart problem was taken care of. He said that he travelled to the state of Uttar Pradesh, where he met up with a very famous 'Baba', who was known to cure all sorts of illnesses. When he explained his case history, the 'Baba' thrust his hand forward and put it through Mr Abdul's chest. He then removed his heart, applied some holy ash on the areas of blockage and put the heart back in. After this 'cure', he had been fine, and was now able to go about his daily activities without any discomfort, and had stopped all his medication.

I was totally speechless, though a battle raged in my head about whether to disabuse him of the notion that he was 'cured', or to let him preserve the fantasy in his head, however false that might be. In the end, I chose the middle path, and congratulated him on his successful cure, but managed to convince him to continue with his heart medication. Since I am a doctor and do not possess the special powers of the 'Baba', I will stick to recommending bypass surgery for such patients, and hope that they feel just as well as Mr Abdul.

Everyone dreads the Big B (no, I am not referring to Amitabh Bachchan) when they have heart disease. When you tell a patient that they require bypass surgery, it almost feels like you have pronounced a death sentence on them. In many ways, nothing could be further from the truth. With the advances in medical science and techniques, it would not be an exaggeration to say that today, a bypass surgery is almost as routine and straightforward as a hernia repair or appendicectomy was a few decades ago. In good surgical centres, the mortality rate is usually under 1 per cent; which means less than one person dies for every 100 operated. The rare surgical deaths that do occur are usually in patients who are in very bad health prior to surgery and often with other medical complications such as kidney failure.

How is it done?

As the name suggests, the goal of the operation is to bypass a blocked artery. Just as a detour is created for the free flow of vehicles on a road on which construction is taking place, a bypass is created for the free flow of blood around the blockage. (Of course, you could never create such a detour on the roads of Mumbai, since the detour too would get choked up immediately!)

The surgeon connects one end of a healthy artery to the coronary artery at an area beyond the blockage. This connecting artery is called a 'bypass graft', hence the official name of the surgery is coronary artery bypass graft (CABG) surgery, commonly referred to as 'cabbage' surgery in some Western countries. The artery most commonly used as a graft is your chest artery known as the left internal mammary artery or LIMA. It is disconnected from one end and stitched to your coronary artery. Often, after making one connection, known as an anastomosis, the LIMA is continued on and further connections are made at different portions below the blockage.

I sometimes joke that the cardiac surgeon is like a very skilful tailor who stitches arteries instead of clothes. Remember that these arteries are about 2 mm in thickness, and then you will realize why your cardiac surgeon and tailor don't have the same income or level of respect!

The LIMA is usually grafted to the LAD and this graft remains open or 'patent' for several decades. The LIMA is the first choice of artery used for grafting, but there are others that can be used when more grafts are needed. The common grafts used are the right internal mammary artery, the radial artery (taken from your arm) and the saphenous vein, taken from your leg. All the early CABG surgeries used saphenous veins as grafts, but it was found that these got blocked within a relatively short period of time, and are not used that often anymore.

Once the grafting is done, the source of blood supply to the area below the blockage comes from the new artery, but the blockage does not go away. Most patients are under the impression that the surgeon opens up the artery, cleans out the plaque, and throws it away (probably in a dustbin), before closing up the artery and the chest wall. Instead, the blockage remains where it has always been, but now becomes irrelevant since your heart has 'new pipes' supplying it with blood. This is probably the reason most patients say that they are 20 years younger after a bypass. I remind them that this is a bypass surgery not a botox surgery, and for them to be younger or even feel younger, they need to work on their lifestyle habits.

What is beating heart surgery?

The coronary arteries run on the surface of the heart, and consequently are constantly moving in rhythm with the beating of the heart. Therefore it is impossible to stitch one artery to another while the heart is moving (remember they are only 2–4 mm thick). To overcome this, doctors invented the heart-lung machine. As the name suggests, this machine temporarily takes over the functions of the heart and lungs and allows the heart to be stopped. While the heart is stopped, the surgeon does the grafting, and the heart is restarted.

Since the last decade, some surgeons are now performing what is known as an off-pump, or 'beating heart surgery'. Again, as the name suggests, the heart continues beating while the grafting is done. An instrument called the Octopus is used to stabilize portions of the heart where the grafting is to be done while the rest of the heart continues beating. This is an extremely complicated procedure which requires even more skill than a regular bypass surgery. The advantage to the patient is that the potential ill-effects of stopping the heart are avoided (you could say they are bypassed!). Some of the negative effects of stopping the heart with the heart-lung machine include short-term memory loss, decline in fine motor skills, and release of small blood clots which may lead to stroke. One of the disadvantages of beating heart surgery is the greater skill requirement of the surgeon, which is why the best surgical results are usually obtained at centres which perform a high number of such surgeries each year.

How many grafts are used for the surgery?

Amitabh Khona is one of the nicest people you can come across. His nephew is a good friend of mine, and asked me to take special care of him after his surgery. Though we live in a city of 15 million people, it's amazing how small it is in many ways. It is not uncommon for a doctor to receive calls from four different sources for each patient, asking them to be taken 'special care' of.

Amitabh was a 57-year-old advertising and PR man, and he looked and played the part. After his surgery, he was chatting with me one day, when he very proudly told me that he held the record for the maximum number of blocks found on an angiography. As you can see, men will be men, and size does matter, even if it's related to disease. He told me that he had 11 blocks, but was confused as to why he needed only seven grafts. Often the number of blocks seen on angiography and the number of grafts differ, and to understand this riddle, think of the plumbing pipes in your building. If a pipe is blocked at the point where it bifurcates to two houses, then both houses will not receive adequate supply and two new channels will need to be created, one to each house. On the other hand, if the pipe is travelling between two floors, then even if there are two blockages along the length, both can be solved by attaching an alternate supply below the lower blockage. In the first example, two new connections (think of them as grafts) were needed for one blockage, while in the second example, two blockages were taken care of by one 'graft'. You may have heard the term 'triple bypass surgery' or 'quadruple bypass' surgery. These terms indicate the number of locations where grafting has been done.

Other open heart surgeries

The term open heart surgery simply suggests that the chest bone is cut open and the heart is operated upon. Bypass surgery is the most frequently performed open heart surgery, but there are other types of open heart surgeries as well. The most common of these is valve surgery, to repair or replace the aortic valve or mitral valve. While the actual surgery differs, the care that needs to be taken by these patients post-surgery remains the same as that for bypass surgery. One difference is their need to take special blood-thinning medications and maintain the 'thinness' of their blood, known as INR, within a certain range.

What to expect after the surgery?

The actual surgery is much easier for the patient than the relatives in many ways. Thanks to the anaesthesia, the patient is blissfully unaware of time, while the relatives are waiting outside the operation theatre biting their nails off. The patient is taken from the operating room to the intensive care unit, where the average length of stay is two to three days. He is then transferred to the wards, where he spends an average of five to six days before being discharged.

Several decades ago, any patient with a heart problem would be restricted to bed, and asked not to move for at least four weeks. All that changed with the publication of a landmark study in 1966, known as the Dallas Bed Rest and Training Study. They took five healthy men who were 20 years old, and made them rest in bed for three weeks. They measured their aerobic exercise capacity before and after bed rest and found a dramatic decrease after bed rest. Thanks to this study, physicians woke up to the deleterious effects of bed rest, and starting prescribing activity much earlier after a heart attack and other illnesses.

Thirty years after the original study, the researchers got back the same five study participants, and their exercise capacity levels were measured. The astonishing finding was that these levels were the same as those experienced after three weeks of bed rest 30 years earlier. In other words, three weeks of bed rest (even at the young age of 20) was equivalent to three decades of aging. Bypass surgery is supposed to make a person 20 years younger, not older, so I encourage my patients to start walking the moment they are in the ward and are clinically stable. Some patients may have complications which may slow down their progress, but most are able to walk for at least a few minutes by the time they are ready to be discharged from the hospital.

The first week at home

Most people are extremely happy to return home after hospitalization. They usually have the whole family waiting for them at the door, and a small pooja ceremony is done before they enter the house. They are relieved to be out of the sterile confines of the hospital ward (and the mounting bills), and to sleep in their own bed. However, for some, there is also a sense of nervousness, since the blanket of security that the hospital provided has now been lifted and they need to fend for themselves. While in hospital, the nurse kept track of the day's events and magically appeared when needed. At home they need to do everything themselves, or to be more accurate, now their families need to do everything for them. I must add, that in my experience, Indian men are extremely dependent on their wives to keep track of their medications and their scheduled times. Unfortunately the reverse is not usually true when the lady is the patient.

In the first few days, even small amounts of activity may make you tired and tasks of daily living which you usually take for granted may seem like a major effort. Do not worry, as this is not unusual. Within a few days, your strength and confidence will return and you should be able to resume most of your home-related activities. When you do feel tired, take a short rest before resuming activity. At the same time, you must not give in to those tired feelings and spend all day in bed. Remember what happened to those five young men in Dallas?

Right amount of rest

It is important to rest between activities. While activity and exercise is very important for your recovery, there is a fine line between the right activity and excessive activity. Often this leads to friction with family members, who believe that the patient must get as much rest as possible, and tend to be overprotective. Just as you plan your activity, it is also important to plan your rest periods. Make sure you get adequate sleep at night for at least seven to eight hours. If you wish to, you may take a short nap every afternoon for the first few weeks, but this is optional.

Aches and niggles

After any major surgery, it is quite common for almost all patients to face minor aches and niggles. To be fair to them, it might seem minor to us as doctors, but the patient sees it differently. When I say minor, it's more to suggest that these are usually short-lived and will not affect the course of recovery.

One thing that has struck me after seeing thousands of patients undergoing serious surgery is how their bowel movement seems to be their most important health concern. I cannot tell you the number of times I have come across patients who are more anguished that they have not 'passed motion' for a day than about any cardiac or neurological issue. I don't know whether this obsession is peculiar to Indian patients or is seen all over the world. As part of the aches and niggles category, some sleep excessively, while others don't sleep at all, some get bouts of diarrhoea, while others are constipated. When they come to me with these complaints, I ask them to be patient, and remind them of the ancient proverb, 'This too shall pass'.

At the same time, if you are experiencing discomfort which is more than mild, don't ignore it. For example, it is normal to experience some itching, soreness or numbness in the chest area, around your incision. However, if you notice swelling, oozing, warmth, or redness around the area, please inform your doctor.

Laughter is the best medicine

Each individual is different, and the other day I came across a most unique patient. Jayesh Rupani is a 48-year-old businessman who lives in Tanzania. He had his bypass surgery with six grafts in March 2013. When I met him four weeks after his surgery he said that everything was fine with him, except that he could not control his laughter after surgery. Ordinarily that would not be a bad thing, except that his chest 'hurt like mad' each time he laughed uncontrollably. I looked at his wife, who corroborated the story, and added that one time he laughed so much he actually fell off the chair, and that wasn't funny.

I reminded him that laughter is the best medicine, and if this was his only complaint post-operatively, then he is a lucky man. He greeted that with a loud laugh, and told me many more interesting stories, some of which are quoted later in the book.

Busting relatives' myths

During a lecture I was taking for post-operative patients, one of them called out my name to get my attention, and then proceeded to ask his question in sign language. This perplexed me, since his voice had sounded perfectly fine a moment ago. When I asked him why he was not speaking, he told me that his relatives had said that he should avoid talking after surgery. This is the most common myth I have heard in my years of practice. For some reason, most relatives strictly instruct their patients not to speak after surgery. There is no scientific explanation for this, and on a lighter note, I wonder if the relatives are just tired of hearing the patient's voice, and need a break!

This reminds me of an interesting consultation I had with a patient and his wife. Sunil Khadye was a 60-year-old engineer of Indian origin living in Dubai. On one of his visits to India, while climbing up to the temple of Ekvira Devi near Pune, he developed chest pain. Subsequent testing revealed triple vessel disease, for which he had a bypass surgery. When I met him and his wife post-surgery, she was silent throughout the meeting and at the end had only one question—when will his voice return to normal? Sometimes after a major surgery, due to tubes being put in the throat, a patient develops hoarseness of voice, and in rare instances, the voice is lowered to a whisper. I assured her that it would be back to normal within two months, but was curious to know why that was the only question she had. She smiled shyly and revealed that his voice was what had captured her attention 30 years ago.

The other issue which comes up is whether to allow visitors once the patient is home. Caregivers normally like to restrict visitors due to the fear of possible infection spreading to the patient. In my opinion, there is nothing wrong with visitors, except for the fact that most of them turn into cardiologists the moment they enter the patient's room and are full of advice on what to do and what to eat. Most of the advice is wrong, and only confuses the patient. In India it's traditional to leave your footwear at the doorstep before entering someone's house. I suggest that visitors should be allowed, but they should be asked to leave their advice at the doorstep too.

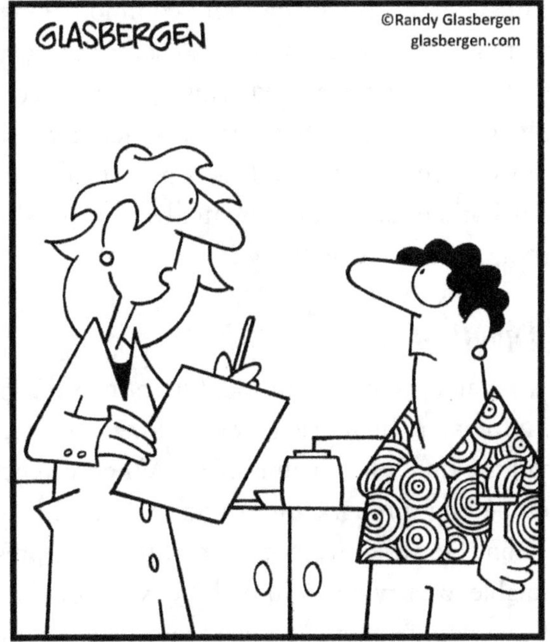

"You have many weight-loss options:
gastric bypass, donut shop bypass,
pizza parlor bypass, buffet bypass..."

Pain after surgery

To perform open heart surgery, the surgeon has to cut open the breast bone, known as the sternum. After surgery, strong wires hold the sternum together and the healing process begins. This takes about six to eight weeks. During this time, it's normal to feel pain, tightness, or a 'pulling' sensation in the chest region. This discomfort may also be felt in the shoulder, neck or back, as well as in the arm, from which an artery has been removed. I explain to my patients that while this is uncomfortable, it is totally normal and not dangerous. This does not make the pain less, but it does make them feel relieved that nothing has gone wrong. If the pain is unbearable you may take painkillers as advised by your doctor. It's also normal to have a slight elevation of the sternum at its upper end, where it protrudes out a little, like a small lump. Patients are usually bothered by this, but it does not cause pain and is harmless. Another common complaint is numbness along the forearm, and in some of the fingers. This is usually more common along the arm from where the radial artery has been taken, but also happens sometimes in an arm from which no artery has been removed. This takes place due to pinching of the nerves supplying sensation to that particular area, and usually goes away after a few months. In some patients it does persist, but rarely limits their daily activities. It bothers them more mentally than physically, and when they start accepting it, it miraculously goes away.

The emotional quotient

Heart surgery is a major event in your life. Oftentimes the gap between the first onset of symptoms and surgery is a short one and in the flurry of activities, you have not had the time to stop and reflect. When you get home, all the emotions come flooding through, and it's normal to sometimes experience bouts of depression. However, it's not normal to feel depressed to a point where you are unable to carry out your daily activities even four to six weeks after surgery. If that does happen, you need to consult your doctor.

Physical activity after surgery

Walking

During your stay in the hospital you will have started a walking program. Exercise improves your strength after surgery and also helps increase your cardiac capacity. During the first week at home, people generally prefer to walk within the house. However, if you would prefer to walk in your building compound or neighbourhood, you may do so.

Below is a sample walking program. There are always individual differences and you need to adjust your program depending on how you feel. Do not worry if you are unable to follow the program exactly. If your ejection fraction is on the lower side (less than 35 per cent), you need to progress on a slower basis—start with three to five minutes the first week and stay on the lower side of the suggested guidelines.

Post-surgery walking program

WEEK NO. (AFTER DISCHARGE)	DURATION (MINS)	TIMES PER DAY
1	5-10	3-4
2	10-15	3-4
3	15-20	2-3
4	20-25	2
5	25-30	1
6	30-45	1

Climbing stairs

For the first few weeks, if there is an elevator available, it is better to use it to reach your destination. If however you do need to climb steps, then you need to do so in a gradual manner. Take a break for 30-60 seconds after every few steps. Listen to your body—if you feel breathless and need to take a longer break, go ahead and do so. After complete recovery it's a good idea to climb steps as part of your everyday activity.

Note: If your ejection fraction is on the lower side (less than 35 per cent), consult your doctor or cardiac rehabilitation specialist before initiating stair climbing.

Lifting Restrictions

As a general guideline, do not lift anything heavier than 3 to 4 kilograms for six weeks after surgery. Heavy lifting can cause the bone in your chest to separate, and prevent it from healing. Avoid pushing/pulling heavy objects, or working with your arms overhead. These activities disproportionately elevate blood pressure and put an added strain on a healing heart.

Driving

You can start driving after six to eight weeks of surgery after consulting with your surgical team/cardiologist. Driving by itself is not a difficult activity, but the fear is the impact against the steering wheel in case of an accident. Depending on the impact, it may lead to a separation of the sutures which are holding the breast bone together. However, you may travel by car immediately after discharge, but please make sure you are wearing your seatbelt at all times.

Getting back to work

The decision on when to resume work depends on a number of factors, including the severity of illness, the nature of work, and the physical health of the person prior to the event. After bypass surgery, it is usually advisable to wait for a period of four to six weeks before resuming work. Another factor, which is most important, is the patient's desire to return to work. It's not uncommon to come across patients in public sector employment who are quite content to make full use of their paid sick leave, and are happy to stay at home for two months (some even ask for longer). On the other hand, you come across Type A personalities who run their own businesses, and sneak below the blanket and work on their iPads even in the ICU!

Other frequently asked questions

It is not an unusual sight to see someone tying a patient's shoelace after bypass surgery. Patients and their relatives have this fear instilled in them that after surgery they should not bend forward at all. In my mind, this fear is greatly exaggerated, and if the patient were to bend forward for a few seconds, there would be no problem. Acts of daily living, such as bending to pick up something on the ground, or leaning forward while brushing your teeth are perfectly fine. The recommendation is not to bend far forward and remain in that position for long. Quite frankly, none of us do that in our daily lives, in any case.

Another question patients have is, will their ejection fraction (EF-pumping capacity) improve after surgery, assuming it was low to begin with. This is a tricky one to answer, and my best reply is 'maybe'. A person's EF is low due to heart muscle damage. Some of the damage is permanent and some temporary. Where the damage is temporary, restoration of better blood supply after the surgery would lead to better functioning and the EF can improve. On the other hand, if the damage is permanent, the EF may remain the same.

Cardiac rehabilitation

A few weeks after a bypass surgery or any major cardiac intervention, it is crucial that the patient enrol in a structured cardiac rehabilitation program. Extensive research has been done which shows that when compared with usual medical care, patients who participate in a cardiac rehabilitation program have a reduction of 20 per cent in total death and 26 per cent in cardiac deaths. In fact, such is the importance, that leading cardiology associations like the American Heart Association have classified it as a Class I (must-do) recommendation, on par with other life-saving measures like a daily aspirin dose. Research has also shown that patients enrolled in a cardiac rehab program had a 47 per cent decreased chance of having a heart attack, compared to those who did not. Getting a surgery done is the first half of your treatment. Getting back to normalcy quickly and safely is the second half, which is as important. In my experience a good cardiac rehab program has great long-term benefits in improving the physical as well as mental health of the patient.

How long does the bypass surgery last?

A common concern shared by patients is how long their bypass surgery will last. Here, I am not talking about how long the actual surgery takes, which is usually between four to eight hours, but I am referring to how long the new grafts will continue functioning effectively. My answer to them is as long as they take good care, and while it sounds simplistic, it's actually the truth. Research has shown that the left internal mammary artery (LIMA) remains patent or open in 90 per cent of cases even after 10 years, and there are several studies showing that they remain open even after 20 years. Other grafts used, such as the saphenous vein and radial artery, do not have quite as good a track record, but with appropriate care, can remain patent for a long time. The majority of responsibility for long-term success is now in your hands. If you are able to follow the lifestyle guidelines suggested in this book, along with regular medical follow-up, there is no reason that you should ever suffer from heart disease again.

Take-home messages

- In a bypass surgery a new artery is connected to the coronary artery below the area of blockage. A detour is created around the blockage—the blockage is not removed.

- The new artery is called a bypass graft, and the left internal mammary artery (LIMA) is most commonly used for this purpose.

- In a beating heart or off-pump surgery, the heart continues beating while the surgeon performs the procedure. In an on-pump surgery, the heart is temporarily stopped, using a heart-lung machine.

- After surgery it is important to get mobile and physically active as soon as possible. Prolonged bed rest is detrimental.

- Cardiac rehabilitation is an integral part of post-surgery care, and will help you recover quickly and safely. You should be able to resume a healthy life within six to eight weeks of surgery.

8

Angioplasty

(Opening up the pipes)

SHYAM SUNDER SURI WAS CONDUCTING A HARD NEGOTIATION IN THE COFFEE shop at the Trident Hotel in the Bandra Kurla Complex in Mumbai when he started feeling uneasy in the stomach, and had to rush to the wash room. Mr Suri was an IIM-A graduate who had founded a successful BPO company that employed 5,000 people. Normally a very calm person, he was quite excitable at the meeting, and the washroom was a welcome break. However, after returning, he found that he was sweating, even though the air-conditioning was on full blast. He knew that something was wrong, and decided to seek medical help. The hotel staff offered to take him to the Asian Heart Institute, which is a stone's throw away. On the way to the elevator he threw up, and suspected that he had some kind of food poisoning. In the car en route to the hospital, his chest started hurting, with the severity increasing by the minute. At the hospital he was diagnosed with an acute inferior wall MI, which meant that the lower portion of his heart had suffered a heart attack. Since he was diagnosed in less than an hour after his pain first started, he was offered the option of a PAMI, which is an angioplasty done during a heart attack (primary angioplasty in myocardial infarction). This proved life-saving for Mr Suri, and within minutes of the procedure, the heaviness was lifted off his chest, and his ECG had come back to normal. He was lucky to have received treatment in time, and his heart muscle was left with no permanent damage.

What is an angioplasty?

An angioplasty—technically known as a percutaneous transluminal coronary angioplasty (PTCA)—is a procedure in which a catheter is threaded through the coronary arteries and passed through the area of blockage. A balloon is then passed over it and inflated at extremely high pressure (6 to 15 times the atmospheric pressure) to push the blockage to the wall of the artery. If you can compare the job of a bypass surgeon to that of a tailor you could say an interventional cardiologist is like a plumber who opens up a blocked pipe.

Traditionally, the catheter was inserted into the femoral artery, with access from the groin, but over the last decade, radial artery access via the wrist has gained popularity. One of the benefits of the radial approach is that the person can be discharged quicker, and can start walking almost immediately after the procedure.

When should you do an angioplasty?

If you are having a heart attack and reach the hospital within 12 hours of the onset of your symptoms, then a PAMI is clearly the best choice of treatment (some studies suggest that it should be done up to 24 hours from the onset of symptoms). That said, the sooner you reach, the better is the outcome, which underscores the importance of getting to a hospital fast, rather than arguing with your spouse, waiting for your family doctor to arrive, and finally reaching the hospital.

However, in other settings, the usefulness of an angioplasty has been questioned, especially in comparison with standard aggressive medical management with drugs and lifestyle changes. In 2009, the American College of Cardiology released guidelines on the 'appropriateness criteria' for revascularization, which includes angioplasty and bypass surgery. These guidelines were again revised in the year 2012. According to these, there are very few situations outside the setting of an acute myocardial infarction in which an angioplasty has proven to be superior to medical management to improve survival. A significant blockage in the early part of the LAD artery is one of these situations. Angioplasty has also been found to be beneficial only in symptom relief for those suffering from angina (and do not feel better even after being on optimal drug therapy). In other words, if you do not have any symptoms, but discovered heart disease by chance, then there is usually no benefit in having an angioplasty done, and in fact there may be harm. These are general guidelines, and each individual situation needs to be assessed keeping the patient's overall health profile in mind. In an audit done in the United States, they found that close to 20 per cent of the angioplasty procedures done were deemed to be inappropriate, using these criteria. I shudder to think what that number is in India, where unlike the US, doctors are not ruled by lawyers and the insurance industry.

Stents

In the past it was found that after doing the angioplasty there was a very high chance of the wall of the artery closing in after the balloon was removed. This closure was seen in about half the number of cases. To reduce this occurrence, scientists designed a stent, which is a small cylindrical tube made out of special metal. After the blockage is opened up with a balloon, the stent is passed through the catheter and left at the site to act as scaffolding.

A stent actually looks like the spring which we used to find around the refills of ball-point pens in the past. It is usually a few millimetres wide and about 15–30 mm long. Today the use of stents has become so common that when we refer to an angioplasty, it usually refers to the balloon plus stent placement.

Your body recognizes a stent as a foreign substance, and sometimes as a defence mechanism generates scar tissue formation inside the artery. This tissue can protrude through the mesh of the stent and encroach upon the lumen and cause narrowing of the artery, known as in-stent restenosis. In simple language we could call it stent failure. The percentage of stent failure was better than the 50 per cent recurrence rates with simple angioplasty, but was still close to 30 per cent. Scientists went back to the drawing board and in the year 2002, introduced polymer or drug-coated stents, known as drug-eluting stents. These are stents covered with different drugs, which are slowly released into the bloodstream to prevent restenosis. Stent failure rates have been drastically cut, but in recently published studies which looked at thousands of these procedures across different centres, they found the average rate was 20 per cent. This is a great reduction from the early days of angioplasty, but in my view is still a very high number.

Stents are a multi-billion dollar industry, and in the quest of making the perfect stent (and maybe some more money), device-manufacturers have now released a biodegradable stent. This stent will dissolve in the body over time, but will continue keeping the artery patent for a much longer period of time. It has been released at the end of 2012, and it's still too early to tell whether it will live up to its promise. Angioplasty without stenting is rarely done these days, and when it is, it's referred to by the rather derogatory sounding term POBA, which stands for 'plain old balloon angioplasty'.

Chances of stent failure

At the time of writing this chapter, I was cycling alongside the Arabian Sea on a pre-dawn winter morning, with my cycling partner and friend Jaideep Khanna. The air felt cold and pure and there was barely any traffic on the roads (believe it or not, that can happen in Mumbai every once in a while). Instead of enjoying the moment, I was obsessing about stents and the probability of restenosis or stent failure. Rather than breaking my head over it, I figured that Jaideep would be the best person to answer a mathematical question, since he is an investment banker and math is his passion. I asked him if the average rate of failure for a stent is 20 per cent, what are the chances that a person with two, three, or four stents might have failure in any one of them? He shot me the same dirty look he usually reserves for speeding cabbies and bus drivers for spoiling his morning ride, but at the same time couldn't resist solving the puzzle. What he told me left me in a state of shock. If you have one stent inserted, then the chance of failure is 20 per cent. If you have two, then the chances that any one of them might fail is 36 per cent; if you have three, the number goes up to 49 per cent; if you have four, this increases to 59 per cent, and if you have five, then it touches a whopping 67 per cent. In other words, if you have five stents, then there are two out of three chances that one of the stents will fail. This is certainly not a very comforting thought, since it is very common these days for multiple stent insertions in patients.

What happens if there is stent failure?

Leena Das was on holiday with her husband in Chennai when she had a heart attack. Luckily she was rushed to the nearest hospital and an angiography was done immediately. It revealed blockages in the LAD and right coronary artery. The blockage in the LAD was the one that had ruptured and caused a heart attack, and was labelled as the 'culprit lesion'. An immediate angioplasty was done for the LAD and three days later another was done for the block in the right coronary artery. She returned to Mumbai, and enrolled in our cardiac rehab program. At the time of starting, she and her husband were both very anxious, since she was only 50 years old, and was very nervous about her future. She was doing well for two months, but then began to experience pain in her jaws after 10 minutes of walking. This pain was consistently brought on by walking and relieved at rest or by taking Sorbitrate. I observed this a few times, and when it did not seem to go away, I recommended her to do an angio. The angio revealed restenosis in the stent in the right coronary artery. Since the block was not in a crucial location, and there was already an instance of stent failure, it was decided to continue her on aggressive medical management and not do a repeat plasty.

If restenosis is to occur, it usually takes place within six months of stent placement. One of the signs of it taking place is your original symptoms returning, such as chest heaviness. When these symptoms return, you may be recommended to undergo a stress test or even an angiography to confirm the diagnosis. The consequences of the restenosis will depend on the degree of blood flow obstructed, and in some cases it could even lead to a heart attack. It will also depend on the location of the original stent. For example, a stent in the early part of the LAD getting blocked again is far more dangerous than the same happening in a small branch of the LAD. The options available include putting in another stent within the original stent, or inserting a balloon and opening it up, or even a bypass surgery in some cases. Sometimes, as in Mrs Das' case, your cardiologist may suggest no intervention, but regular medical follow-up.

Going home after angioplasty

Usually the patient spends the first night after an angioplasty in the ICU, and is discharged the next day or the day after that. This will also depend on the medical condition of the patient prior to the procedure. If it was a case of PAMI, then the patient may be kept in the hospital for a few days longer, under observation.

Compared to a bypass surgery, an angioplasty is far less invasive and patients are able to start home activities almost as soon as they return. Once they are home they can begin a walking program as described below:

Post-angioplasty walking program

Week no.	Duration (mins)	Times per day
1	5-10	3-4
2	10-15	3-4
3	20-30	2
4	30-45	1

Getting back to normalcy

Most patients want to know when they will be normal again. I always find that question amusing since, for most of them, normal means leading a very sedentary life, and not being particularly careful of their diet, or lifestyle habits. So when they ask me that question, I sometimes reply, 'Never.' I wait for a second for a look of horror to spread over their face, before I smile and quickly reply, 'You will be better than normal,' and they are immediately reassured. (I learned this little game from my daughter: every time I asked her if she loves daddy, she would say no. And then she would see the sad look on my face, and say she doesn't just love her daddy, she adores him.)

After an angioplasty you can resume driving and get back to work within a week, provided there were no complications after the procedure, and you have not had a recent heart attack. If the plasty was preceded by a heart attack, then it is usually recommended to wait four to five weeks before resuming work.

Medication after angioplasty

To reduce the rate of restenosis, the patient is prescribed two types of blood-thinning medications: aspirin and clopidogrel (or prasugrel). Different cardiologists like to continue dual therapy for different lengths of time, but the recommendation is to prescribe both for at least a period of a year. These help to prevent stent failure, and it is vital that for the first year both these medications be taken without missing a single day. Besides these, you also need to take your routine medications for heart disease, which we will talk about in-depth in the chapter on medications.

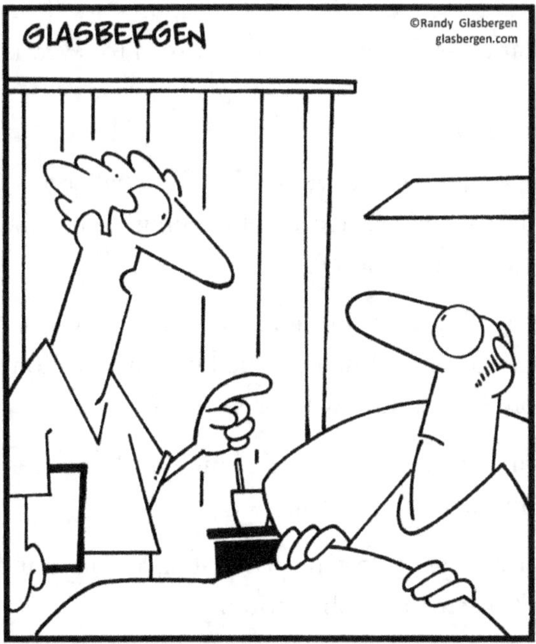

"First we insert a balloon to open the clogged artery, then we fill the balloon with helium so you weigh less."

Cardiac Rehabilitation

As I had recommended after bypass surgery, it is important that you enrol in a structured cardiac rehabilitation program after angioplasty too. It will help you get back to a healthy way of life very quickly and safely. In most cases, it can be started within a week of your plasty. Since most patients remain in hospital only for a few days for their plasty, they tend to 'feel' normal very quickly, and tend to ignore the importance of long-term care. This is a big mistake and is often the reason we see the same patient coming back to us after a few years, with a problem in some other artery. Nobody wants to have a repeat heart procedure, but if you truly want to prevent it and try to reverse the disease process, then you need to work hard at it, and good cardiac rehabilitation is the first step on the road to reversal.

Take-home messages

- In an angioplasty (also known as PTCA), a balloon is inflated at high pressure at the site of blockage. After opening the block, a stent is usually placed there to keep the artery open.

- A stent is a small, cylindrical, metal object which acts as scaffolding to keep the artery patent. Most are coated with medication, which prevents the stent from closing (known as restenosis).

- Restenosis or stent failure can be as high as 20 per cent and it usually occurs within the first six months.

- After angioplasty, it's important to maintain a healthy and active lifestyle, and to enrol in cardiac rehabilitation.

9

Reversal of Heart Disease

(Turning back the clock)

CHANDRESHEKAR SAWANT IS A LEAN 57-YEAR-OLD BUSINESSMAN WHOSE athletic body looks like he might break into a run any time. Looking at him, one would find it hard to believe that, in December 2009, he was lying on a surgical table with a catheter in his groin, just having completed an angiography.

It is cold in the cath lab at 18 degrees centigrade, but it feels colder when the doctor is about to pronounce the outcome of your angiogram. Like a judge announcing his verdict, the outcome has the potential of dramatically altering your life. His doctor told him that he had blockages in all three of his heart arteries, and suddenly Mr Sawant felt that he had been transported to the Arctic Circle and was lying in the snow without his clothes. Prior to his angiography, he had done a thallium stress test, which was abnormal after 7 minutes and 41 seconds of exercise. He was advised an angioplasty in two of his arteries, and to leave the third alone for the moment. That's when Mr Sawant decided that he wanted to leave all three of them alone, not just for the moment, but forever.

When he met me, I felt that the blocks were not critical, and it would be appropriate to put him on what is known as 'medical management'. Medical management basically implies that we are not doing an angioplasty or bypass surgery on the person. He enrolled in our cardiac rehab program and made serious lifestyle changes, which included exercise, dietary modification and stress management. After three years, Mr Sawant went back for a thallium stress test. This time he did 13 minutes and 21 seconds, which is a better result than most healthy 30-year-olds can achieve. And what is more, there were no ECG changes, and the test was labelled as normal. In 2009, his cardiologist had written on his prescription note, 'Avoid undue exertion'. In 2013, Mr Sawant ran a half marathon! Had he reversed heart disease? Did his blockages just get dissolved and flushed away?

Can heart disease really be reversed?

I am asked this question or some variant of it nearly every day in my clinic, and I really do not have a simple answer. The reason why there isn't an easy answer to this question has to do with the nature of the disease, and the nature of the cure.

As has been explained in earlier chapters, your coronary arteries are like pipes which supply blood to your heart muscle. The process of blockage development, or atherosclerosis, takes place over a number of years, often over decades. It slowly increases in size and blocks a portion of the opening within the artery, compromising blood flow to your heart muscle. The blockage contains a number of 'junk substances' including cholesterol, calcium and dead blood cells. The more cholesterol it contains, the 'softer' is the plaque (another word for the blockage), and the more unstable it is. As it progresses, one of two scenarios are likely to occur.

1. The plaque progresses slowly and occludes more of the lumen of the artery, and over time this usually gives rise to some symptoms of angina. While this is growing steadily, the heart senses the lack of blood supply, and begins to develop 'collaterals'. These can be looked upon as newer blood vessels, which provide alternate channels for blood supply to the heart muscles. The slower the disease progresses, greater the chance of collateral formation. When an angio is performed in such a case, it is not surprising for the original blockage to even be 100 per cent. Patients often wonder how they survived with a 100 per cent blockage, and the answer to that is collateral formation. These are usually 'stable' plaques which do not rupture and lead to sudden heart attacks. Rather, they give symptoms of angina, which alert people to get further testing and take appropriate steps.

2. It is also possible that at some point during its growth, the plaque ruptures and causes the formation of a thrombus, or blood clot, which shuts off blood supply to a part of the heart muscle. Depending on the extent of heart muscle supplied by the shut-off artery, the attack may be minor or major, which could be the difference between survival and death.

3. Therefore, it can be argued that the size of the block may not be as relevant as the stability of the block. In other words, if we manage to keep the person symptom-free and the block 'stable' throughout the person's life, then the size and extent of the block is irrelevant. The whole purpose of this long explanation is to drive home the point that with intensive lifestyle modification and medical management, the stability of the plaque is greatly increased, and the risk of heart attack and death is greatly reduced.

Evidence of reversal

In 1990, a landmark study called the Lifestyle Heart Trial was published by Dr Dean Ornish and his team, which showed that with intensive lifestyle changes it is possible to 'reverse' heart disease. In this study, they divided patients into two groups: one which followed intensive lifestyle changes and the other followed 'usual care'. Angiographies were done before the program and a year later (and also five years later in a follow-up study). The results showed that in the group that followed lifestyle changes, the average blockage percentage had reduced from 40 per cent to 37.8 per cent, and when they looked only at blockages which were greater than 50 per cent, they had reduced from 61.1 per cent to 55.8 per cent. On the other hand, in the usual care group (which is known as the control group in medical studies), the blockages had progressed by about 4 per cent.

In two other important studies, one done at Stanford University and the other in Heidelberg, Germany, researchers looked at before and after angiograms in patients following intensive lifestyle changes versus usual care. Here it must be mentioned that usual care refers to the routine standard of care that is being offered in that particular city at that particular point in time. Over time, as more information is available, interventions which were once considered experimental become usual care too. In both of the studies mentioned above, researchers found that in the lifestyle change groups, the blockages did not change in size over a four to six year period, while in the control group, they increased slightly. However, what is interesting in all of these studies is that the frequency of hospitalizations, heart attacks and other adverse events were greatly reduced in the lifestyle groups.

Physiological reversal takes place

Just like a politician, I have not answered the original question, 'Does reversal take place?', but I promise you I will. What is obvious from these and other studies is that significant reduction in the size of the blockages does not happen even with the most aggressive lifestyle changes and medications. However, these changes lead to two important outcomes. First, the progression of the blockage is usually halted or slowed down significantly. Remember, heart disease is a chronic progressive disease, and therefore the natural course of action is for the blockages to keep increasing. Second, and more importantly, the plaques are stabilized, which in turn prevents them from rupturing and leading to heart attacks.

So, to get to the answer, here is my final take on the subject of reversal of heart disease. I would say that 'physiological' reversal of heart disease does take place, but 'anatomical' reversal does not take place. In other words, the size of the block may not really change, but the chances of heart attack and death greatly reduce and your ability to lead a normal healthy life greatly increases. Now, does that answer the question, or is it still a political answer?

The reversal program

Now that we have established that physiological reversal is possible, the big question is, how does one do it? The reversal program essentially consists of four important pillars, which are exercise, nutrition, medication and stress management. The goal is to aim at aggressive risk factor reduction through lifestyle change, which will in turn reduce the risk of heart attack and death. As I have said several times before, it's like driving a car—the more careful we are, the less the chances of having an accident. Also, there is a difference between getting the numbers within normal range and reducing them to a point which leads to reversal. The classic example is your cholesterol: most doctors will be happy if your LDL cholesterol is near-about 100 mg/dl, but for aggressive reversal you should aim for it to be below 70 mg/dl.

Reversal versus intervention

Not everyone with heart disease needs to have an angioplasty or bypass surgery. In fact, a very small percentage of patients with a diagnosis of heart disease need these procedures. However, every patient (whether they have had an intervention or not) needs to follow a lifestyle program in order to reduce future risk. In other words, they need to follow the principles of what we have called the 'reversal program'. There are some patients who actually need a surgery or angioplasty and refuse to undergo one. It becomes challenging to address this group. As a doctor, it is my duty to offer them the best advice possible, but it is up to the individual to actually follow the advice. If they are insistent on avoiding surgery or plasty, I inform them about the risks in a candid manner, and then leave the choice to them.

Different paths to the reversal program

Essentially, the reversal program is a heart-healthy way of life. This really applies to each and every individual in society, even the very young. In 1953, during the Korean war, autopsies were conducted on American soldiers who had died during combat. In a study that looked at 300 soldiers, it was found that a vast majority of them, 77 per cent to be precise, had at least the early stages of atherosclerosis in their coronary arteries. Their average age was 22! In other words, you are never too young to suffer, and need to initiate these changes as early in life as possible.

For the purpose of easy understanding, let's divide everyone into four broad categories, ranging from those who have heart disease to those who want to prevent it.

1. Those with a recent event, such as a heart attack, angioplasty or bypass surgery

These patients are often the easiest to work with and are most compliant to changes that we recommend them. Since they have suffered recently, they usually want to do everything it takes to get back to normalcy and make sure they never need to go through the heartache again.

2. Heart disease, without an intervention

These are patients who have been diagnosed with heart disease, as seen by angiography or an advanced physiological test, such as a stress echo or stress thallium, but are not in need of an intervention, and have not had a heart attack.

Rajendra Jhaveri was 53 years old when he had a heart attack. He had a strong family history of heart disease, and during the treadmill test he had some chest discomfort and ECG changes and the test was labelled positive. A subsequent angiogram revealed triple vessel disease, for which his cardiologist recommended three angioplasties, or a bypass surgery. Rajendra was not comfortable with the thought of having so much metal in his arteries, or being cut open, so he went in for a second opinion. He was told that he had a chance of averting surgery temporarily provided he made intensive lifestyle changes. I met Rajendra for the first consult in August 2003, and he came across as someone who was determined to avoid surgery as far as possible. I am happy to inform you that it is now 11 years since his angiography, and he is doing wonderfully well in his new life, and has run all 11 Dream Runs of the Standard Chartered Mumbai Marathon. Patients belonging to this category also tend to be motivated and stick to the advice you give them, since they are avoiding a procedure.

3. Risk factors, but no heart disease… yet

These are individuals that have several risk factors for heart disease, but have not been formally diagnosed as 'heart patients'.

Ravi Chawla was 43 years old when he came to me for his routine health check. He was a mid-level manager in an IT company, and led a sedentary life. The only games he played were on the computer, and he jokingly referred to himself as a cyber athlete. His blood pressure was 136/84 mmHg; his total cholesterol was 244 mg/dl; and he was about 6 kilos overweight. All in all, he represented the typical white-collar Mumbaikar. On the stress test his time was 8 minutes and 30 seconds, and it was negative (once more let me remind you that 'negative' means normal). As I was explaining his risk factor profile, he really had only two questions for me: 'Is my stress test normal, and do I need to start any medication?' I assured him that his stress test was fine, but he did have a few risk factors, which included borderline high BP, cholesterol, being overweight and leading a sedentary lifestyle. However, at these levels he did not need medication as all of the above values could be brought under control with lifestyle changes. I then asked for his previous reports and noticed that he had done three health checks over the past five years, and all the values were very similar to the ones he had today.

Ravi's case is more the rule than the exception. Most people have borderline high values on several different risk factors, which they do not take seriously and end up lingering like this for years. Then one fine day, they have a heart attack and wonder how that could have happened when all along the doctor at the annual health check said that they were fine. In such instances I actually tell my patients that instead of borderline values, I wish that their values were high. I wish that the blood pressure, instead of 140/90 was 180/100, and their cholesterol, instead of 244 was 300 mg/dl. Before they think I am mad, I explain that when values are borderline, both the doctor and patient tend to take them lightly. Lifestyle changes are made for a few weeks, and then forgotten. In that manner, borderline values keep continuing for years. They cause mayhem inside the arteries insidiously and one day the perfect storm occurs and you suffer a massive myocardial infarction. You can compare borderline high-risk factors with a very patient prisoner attempting a jailbreak. If the prisoner takes a spoon and tries to burrow a hole in the wall, he will not manage to break the wall in a day, month, or even a year. However, if he persists doing it for 10 years, then he will probably succeed in creating a hole in the wall and a tunnel to escape. Similarly, borderline high BP and cholesterol will not affect your arteries in a day, month, or even a year. But when they continue to be borderline for 10 years and longer, they can cause some serious damage. On the other hand, if your numbers were high instead of borderline, it would be a different scenario. If your cholesterol was 300, or BP was 180, you would be started on pills the same day and would be closely monitored till the numbers came down. You would also be more likely to make and stick to lifestyle changes, if you were keen to get off the pills. It is an irony that patients with higher numbers may be better taken care of and suffer less than those with borderline numbers.

4. Those with optimal risk factor control

This is the easy group. They are the ones who need to be patted on the back and told to carry on doing what they are doing. Unfortunately, there is not much patting to do, since this is a very small group. Optimal risk factor control implies BP below 120/80, total cholesterol below 200 mg/dl, fasting sugar below 100 mg/dl, and a healthy BMI. Of course, it also goes without saying that the person should not be a smoker and should be exercising regularly.

Hold back the invading enemy

To sum it up, think of heart disease as an invading army, which keeps moving forward every day. Think of the reversal program as the defending army. If the defending army is stronger that the one invading, then we will succeed in pushing back the invasion and keep heart disease at bay. It's a long war, in which a few battles may be won by the attacker, but as long as we keep fighting back, long-term success will be ours, and we will be rid of heart disease. The soldiers of our army are all the positive changes that we make through exercise, nutrition and stress management. The rest of the book will talk about how to make these soldiers stronger to better fight the enemy known as heart disease.

Take-home messages

- Heart disease is a progressive disease, which increases with time.

- Intensive lifestyle changes, which involve exercise, nutrition and stress management, have shown to reduce the risk of future heart attacks and death.

- These changes have not shown to decrease the size of the blocks significantly, but have made them more stable, preventing heart attacks.

- With intensive lifestyle changes, physiological reversal of heart disease takes place, more than anatomical reversal.

10

Exercise for the Reversal Program

(The best medicine)

WHEN DHANANJAY YELLURKAR CROSSED THE FINISH LINE OF THE 2012 Mumbai Marathon after running 42.2 gruelling kilometres, there were 75 other smiling heart patients waiting to greet him. They had just completed the Dream Run, and were waiting to welcome their first among equals. He was one of them, and had gone on to prove that heart disease was not the end of life. Actually, the irony is that most of these patients were running because they had heart disease and not in spite of it. Dhananjay and several others had never run long distances in their life, and if it were not for their heart attack, they never would.

However, one does not need to run a marathon to prevent or reverse heart disease. The beauty of exercise as therapy is that you do not need too much of it. Of course, that is not a problem for most people, since their concern is 'how little' they can get away with!

Exercise is medicine

Exercise is the best therapy for prevention and reversal of heart disease. Today there is an entire movement in the United States known as Exercise is Medicine, and physicians are encouraged to write very specific prescriptions for exercise, much the same way they would for medications. It was at one of the Exercise is Medicine annual meetings I attended that a doctor spoke of the discovery of a new wonder drug. He went on to outline the numerous benefits of the drug for heart disease, stroke, diabetes, cancer, osteoporosis, depression and even Alzheimer's disease. Just when the audience's curiosity was at its peak, he turned to the next slide, which was a pair of shoes. The wonder drug is exercise, and all it costs is a pair of shoes. Frankly, with the latest trend towards barefoot running, maybe you don't even need those! All you need are your legs, and your heart.

Exercise has proven to be effective in preventing most chronic diseases suffered by man. Not only does it have these preventive benefits, but for most of these conditions it has therapeutic properties too. It should be part of every doctor's prescription.

Exercise and heart disease

I think it would be safe to say that if you have bought this book and read it this far, I don't need to convince you about the benefits of exercise for heart disease. Exercise has both direct and indirect benefits in reducing heart disease risk. Through exercise, most of the modifiable risk factors can be better controlled. It helps lower your blood pressure, diabetes, cholesterol and body weight, which is how it indirectly helps in reducing heart disease. Besides these, exercise has a direct effect on the functioning of the heart, and allows it to work more efficiently over a longer period of time. With regular exercise, your heart rate at rest is reduced, but the amount of blood pumped during each beat actually increases. In simple words, your heart pumps more efficiently. Besides this, regular exercise causes your blood to become 'less sticky', which is beneficial in preventing a clot (thrombus) which leads to a heart attack. It also modifies the release of some hormones such as adrenaline, and conditions your heart to better deal with emergencies arising out of abnormal heart rhythms.

Dr Carlton Pereira is a young ENT surgeon whom I know well, and when I saw him after a gap of a year, I could barely recognize him. Earlier, he was on the heavy side, and now he looked like a lean, mean fighting machine. I was curious as to why and how he had lost weight, so I asked him. 'I did a lipid profile and my triglycerides were over 600 mg/dl, 631 to be precise. That was about a year ago, and it frightened the hell out of me.

I was advised to start medication, but I was determined to get the values under control through exercise,' was his answer. Triglycerides should ideally be below 150mg/dl, and levels over 600 are clearly dangerous. If he were my patient, I would have insisted that he start medication and continue lifestyle modification simultaneously, but then as the saying goes, 'Doctors never make good patients.'

Carlton embarked on a serious exercise program, where he jogged four times a week, for 40 minutes each, and in a span of six months he lost about 10 kg. His triglycerides showed an improvement, and this spurred him on further. He took up running in a big way, and over the last six months had completed four half-marathons, and was feeling on top of the world. In total, he lost more than 15 kg, and what's more impressive is that his triglycerides dropped a massive 400 plus points, and were now 215 mg/dl.

Exercise is very potent in reducing triglycerides, as well as raising the good HDL cholesterol levels. In the Indian setting that's very important, since we have a tendency to have low HDL levels and high triglycerides. It's safe to say that Dr Pereira is now a lifelong runner and preaches it to all of his patients, whether they come for a sore throat, a nasal polyp, or an ear infection!

The exercise prescription

Since 'exercise is medicine', the amount of exercise recommended should be called the exercise prescription. Rather than view it as a daily prescription, it would make more sense to look at how much exercise should be done per week. At this point it is also important to distinguish between lifestyle physical activity and structured exercise.

Physical activity is any bodily movement which requires energy. Therefore every time you walk from one room to another in your house, it's physical activity. Lifting your fork to your mouth is physical activity—and unfortunately the only physical activity for many. On the other hand, exercise can be defined as physical activity done in a structured manner, with intent to improve health and fitness. Often there is a fine line between physical activity and exercise. For example, if you walked to your office and it took you 10 minutes that would classify as physical activity. But if you went by a longer route and it took you 25 minutes (and you did it at a brisk pace), then it would qualify as exercise.

For most sedentary people, getting off the couch is the first step, and is often the hardest step. When we give detailed exercise prescriptions with precise heart rate guidelines, I have often seen people getting overwhelmed, and they end up doing nothing. Which is why my initial advice to those who are doing nothing at present is to simply start doing *something*. That 'something' could be a daily walk for 10 minutes. Only 10 minutes! Most people laugh and say that's very easy, and I tell them that's all they need to do to get started. Once they achieve this for a whole week, we can take the next step.

Let's get physically active first

Consider daily physical activity as the base of your lifestyle pyramid. Structured exercise sessions should be built on this base and not the other way around. Physical activity includes almost anything we do during the day, except for sitting still and sleeping. In fact, well-documented research has actually shown that those of us who are more fidgety tend to be lighter and fitter than others. The best examples we have in front of us are children. It's fascinating to watch them, especially before the age of 10. My daughter has recently turned 11, and ever since she could walk, I rarely remember her 'walking' in the house. Each time she sets off on a task, she actually runs from room to room. Contrast that with adults, for whom getting up from the sofa to get a glass of water can be a task, and we would rather turn to the domestic help to do it for us. Most adults, once they reach middle age, will lament how their metabolism has slowed down. They will tell you that once upon a time they could eat anything and lose weight at will and now it's so difficult. My theory is that somewhere along our development, we have lost our sense of childhood and physical activity as well as our ability to stop eating when the body is adequately nourished (more of that later, when we talk about food).

Ways to get more active

While it sounds easy enough in theory to increase physical activity, in practice it's much harder. As we have become more industrialized as a nation, the need for physical activity has decreased. Today most people have desk jobs and cars to ferry them to and from their offices. Even homemakers have more help in terms of both domestic workers as well as machines to help make housework much easier. It would not be an exaggeration to say that we now need to get creative to find ways to get physically active. Personally, two methods which work for me are using the stairs, and parking the car further away. At the hospital I used to work at, my department was shifted from the first to the sixth floor. Most of my staff members grumbled that now it took longer to get to work, since they had to stand in queue for the elevator. I saw it as an opportunity to increase my physical activity and continued using the steps. A good rule you can make for yourself is to avoid the elevator as far as possible.

People often ask me if stair climbing is good exercise. I do not recommend it as an exercise, which means I do not suggest that you spend 30 minutes non-stop going up and down the stairs as a substitute for walking or cycling. The reason being that, when done in this continuous manner, it puts undue strain on your joints and may lead to injury over time. On the other hand, I do recommend it strongly as part of your daily physical activity. Each time you need to go up and down a building, use the steps as far as it's practical. Of course, common sense must prevail—I don't expect you to walk up 20 floors each time if you live or work in a high-rise building.

The other trick I use to get in more activity is to park the car slightly away from my final destination. I find that this has a double benefit. Firstly, I get in few extra steps, and more importantly it gives me peace of mind. In Mumbai, where parking is a nightmare, most people will keep circling and getting frustrated till they find the perfect spot very close to the movie hall or restaurant. On the other hand, the moment I am within a half kilometre of where I need to be, I look for a spot. When I do find one, I park my car, and happily walk past the row of frustrated drivers. Try it, and you will realize that even in this crowded city where everyone complains of no parking, you will get by just fine. And, true to my Parsi roots, I avoid giving the car to the valet driver as far as possible.

Airports are another area where one can squeeze in physical activity without realizing it. Fliers spend at least half an hour in the waiting lounge. Instead of fretting and fuming at the invariably delayed flights, it's a great opportunity to walk up and down and get in some bonus activity for the day.

Manish Choudhary is the CFO of a large multinational corporation. I met him during his annual health check, and asked about his physical activity. Being a CFO, I imagined him to be chained to his desk, number crunching all day long. He surprised me when he told me that whenever he went through financial reports (which I imagine must be very often), he did it while standing. He said that he took inspiration from his global boss in New York, who uses a 'standing' desk, and uses bar stools in his office. The bar stools are to encourage a person to sit upright, before you get any ideas.

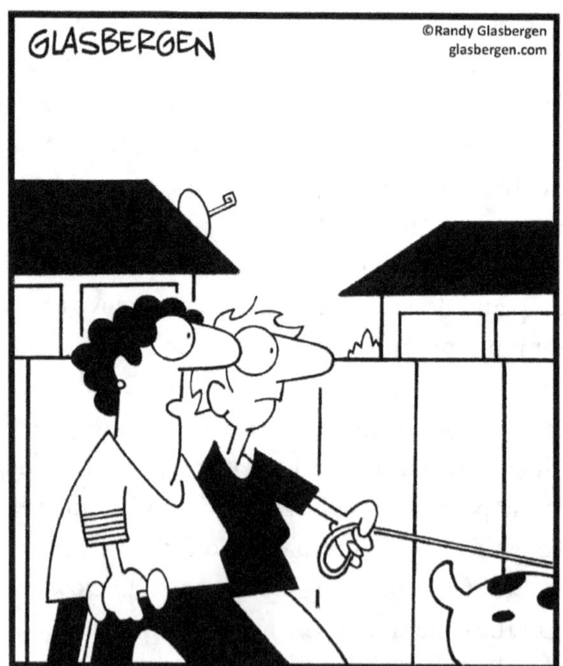

"The doctor told my husband to double his daily exercise, so now he changes channels with both hands!"

Every step counts – get a pedometer

Some of you may be wondering if there really is any benefit in trying to get in these small bouts of physical activity. As the saying goes, every drop makes the ocean, so does each bit of activity contribute to your overall health. Imagine each step you take as putting five rupees in your health savings account. By itself, five rupees is not worth much today, but if you had to deposit it several hundred times a day, for several months and for several years, it would amount to a lot. On the other hand, an exercise session can be seen as a hundred rupee deposit at one time, but it's hard to do that several times a day.

A great tool to monitor your physical activity is a pedometer. It's a small device which clips on to your belt and is about the size of a pager (remember, we used those before cell phones took over our lives). It counts the number of steps you take by sensing your hip movement. For good health, it is recommended that adults take 10,000 steps a day. This roughly translates to walking around 8 km. The good news is that each step is counted, whether it's walking to the wash room, or walking briskly for exercise. I have personally been wearing one for the past six years, and believe me it acts like your conscience sitting on your belt. One person who is clearly happy with this is my wife. Ordinarily it would take a lot of cajoling and coaxing on her part to get me to run small household errands, but now thanks to the pedometer, I am happy to do them and ready for more. I get the benefit of achieving my goal of 10,000 steps, as well as credit from my wife (which as most husbands know, is not an easy thing).

In my opinion, for a few hundred rupees, a pedometer is the best investment you can make for your health. However, it will only work if you use it. Make sure it's clipped to your waist every morning as you leave for work. Remember the famous American Express cards tag line—Don't leave home without it!

10,000 is the magic number

Since most of you may not have used a pedometer, you probably have no clue as to how many steps you currently take in a day. Most executives who have office based jobs, and use their own vehicles for travel, do not do more than 3,000 steps a day, and some may not even touch 2,000. I would suggest using a pedometer for a week and recording your daily steps without worrying too much about the number. Once you have a fair idea about your daily count, set a target which is about 20 per cent higher than your current average. Once you hit that you can keep raising the bar, till you reach the magic figure of 10,000. Make a rule for yourself that you will not go to bed without hitting your daily target. If need be, you can walk after dinner (indoor or outdoor, but at a relaxed pace) to meet your number. The only excuse you should accept for not hitting your target is illness. That's a real reason, all else are just excuses!

The FITT principle of exercise training

Now that you have become a physically active person (hopefully), it's time to add structured exercise to your weekly routine. Broadly, exercise can be divided into cardiovascular training (often abbreviated in gym talk as 'cardio') and strength training. As the name implies, cardio is done to enhance the heart and vascular (blood vessels) system. It is also referred to as aerobic training. Earlier the term aerobics conjured up images of young, fit women dressed in tights, jumping up and down to fast music. Simply put, aerobics refers to any activity which uses oxygen, and is done in a continuous rhythmical manner, such as walking, jogging, cycling, swimming, etc. Decades of research have shown this type of exercise to be very beneficial for the body, especially the heart. The FITT principle refers to the variables we have in our training program.

- F – Is for frequency – how often you should exercise
- I – Is for intensity – how hard you should exercise
- T – Is for time – how many minutes the exercise session should last
- T – Is for the type of exercise

Frequency

Over time there have been different guidelines suggested on how often one must exercise, and they can seem very confusing. One reason is that the total quantum of exercise done over a week can have many permutations and combinations. To keep it simple, I suggest aiming for a total of 150 minutes of moderate intensity exercise per week as a short-term goal (the next three months). You can break this up in any manner, but you should exercise at least three days a week. Once you are comfortable with this routine, you can aim to increase the total duration to 250-300 minutes per week. If you are doing vigorous exercise, such as running or playing squash, then you can get the same benefits in about half the time. When doing vigorous exercise, take at least two days off every week, to give your body recovery time.

Vigorous and moderate exercise is differentiated by the intensity level. During vigorous exercise, your breathing will be much harder, and your heart rate will be significantly faster as exercise intensity increases.

Intensity

I am fortunate to live near the sea in Mumbai, and Marine Drive is my favourite location for a run. My friend Jaideep Khanna was my running partner, and he had only one level of intensity—full on! Clearly he was not familiar with the concept of slowly easing into a run, and keeping up with him used to be a hard task.

When running on Marine Drive, we'd often come across people who would be jogging very slowly and then would suddenly zip past us at high speed. We called them the '100-metre wonders', and would take turns betting how long they would last before abruptly stopping. Intensity is inversely proportional to duration, and the harder you exercise, the shorter you will last, as demonstrated by these 'wonders'.

On the other hand when we ran at the race course, we'd come across middle-aged men walking four abreast and blocking the entire path. Running past them was quite a task. Their speed was so slow we'd wonder if they got any aerobic benefit at all. To gain maximum benefit, you need to exercise at an optimum intensity. The intensity of exercise can be measured in a few different ways:

1. Heart rate guidelines

As you exercise, your heart rate increases. This helps your heart pump more blood per minute to meet the demands of the exercising muscles. At rest, your heart typically pumps out five litres of blood each minute; this is known as the cardiac output. At peak exercise this may increase four to five fold. Increase in heart rate during exercise is a normal phenomenon and should not get you worried. To get maximum cardiovascular benefit, your heart rate during exercise should be between 60–85 per cent of your maximum (max) heart rate.

How to calculate your max heart rate? Your max heart rate (HR) can be calculated using this formula:

$$HR\ (max) = 220 - your\ age$$

This is an estimate, since each and every person's true max cannot be predicted by a common formula. Your true max heart rate can be measured by performing a stress test, in which you push yourself to the point where you cannot sustain exercise even for a few seconds longer. Your heart rate at that point is your true HR max.

While exercising, your heart rate should be between 60–85 per cent of your max. This is known as your target heart rate zone. Research has shown that your body and heart gets maximum aerobic benefit when you exercise in this zone. For some people, it may be difficult to achieve 60 per cent of their heart rate at first, since they may get fatigued before that. Don't worry if that happens, just exercise at a comfortable pace. Over time, you will be able to progress and exercise at a higher intensity. On the other hand, occasionally your heart rate on the upper end may exceed 85 per cent for a few minutes. Do not worry about that either. Exercising at a high rate for a few minutes is not dangerous, but it will be difficult to sustain. There is no fixed cut-off point, but exercise over 80 per cent is generally considered vigorous.

One important point to remember is that several patients take beta-blocker drugs. These are commonly used for high blood pressure and for heart disease. These drugs tend to reduce your heart rate at rest and during max exercise. Therefore the target heart rate zone may not be applicable to those on these medications. If you are taking these drugs, then the RPE scale would be a better method of monitoring intensity. Refer to the table below to see what your heart rate should be at different exercise intensities, depending on your age.

Case Study: Calculate the target heart rate for a 55-year-old person

- Step 1: Find out his HR max on a recently performed stress test. If this is not available, calculate his predicted HR max.
- Predicted HR max = 220 – 55= 165 beats / minute
- Step 2: 60 per cent of his HR max = 165 x .6 = 99 beats / minute
- Step 3: 85 per cent of his HR max = 165 x .85 = 140 beats / minute
- Step 4: His target HR zone is 99 to 140 beats / minute

To measure your heart rate during exercise is extremely difficult, unless you are on a stationary cycle. The best way to do it is to stop exercise for a few seconds and immediately start counting. Count for 15 seconds and multiply the answer by four.

By counting only for 15 seconds, you do compromise a little on accuracy, but if you count longer your heart rate will rapidly start dropping (back towards your resting value). Many exercise machines in the gym have a metal strip, which, when gripped, gives your heart rate reading. I am not sure of their accuracy, though. A heart rate monitor is a better option. It consists of a strap you wear around your chest and a watch on your wrist. The chest strap conveys your heart rate reading to the watch on a continuous basis.

Patients often ask me which the best model is. In my experience, all of them do the job of counting your heart rate well. The more advanced ones also calculate other fitness parameters, such as calories, and allow you to directly download the information to your computer. If you are keen on closely monitoring your exercise parameters, I would highly recommend investing in one.

	Target zone (beats/min)			
Age (yrs)	60 per cent	70 per cent	85 per cent	90 per cent
20	120	140	170	180
25	117	137	166	176
30	114	133	162	171
35	111	130	157	167
40	108	126	153	162
45	105	123	149	158
50	102	119	145	153
55	99	116	140	149
60	96	112	136	144
65	93	109	132	140
70	90	105	128	135
75	87	102	123	131
80	84	98	119	126
85	81	95	115	122

2. RPE scale

A subjective way to measure your exercise intensity is to use a rating of perceived exertion (RPE) scale. This is also called the Borg scale, named after Dr Gunnar Borg of Sweden who invented it in 1959. As the name suggests, it's meant to measure how hard you feel you are exercising.

During exercise, you need to rate your exertion as a number or phrase on the scale (as shown in the figure). Remember, there is no wrong or right answer, it's how you actually feel, and you are the best judge of that. You need to take into account how your entire body feels, and not focus only on your breathing or your muscles. If you are sitting and reading this book, your score should be somewhere close to seven, or very very light (hopefully this book is exercising your grey cells, but here we are only rating physical exertion). On the other hand if you are being chased down by a wild animal, or are sprinting to catch a local train in Mumbai, your exertion level will be upwards of 17, or very hard. On the RPE scale you should maintain a level of 'fairly light to somewhat hard' (11–13) during the major portion of your exercise. For a short duration, you may push the exertion level to 15 (hard), but should return to a lower level before you reach fatigue. Remember that exercise intensity and duration are inversely proportional. That is, the harder you exercise, the shorter the time you will be able to sustain it.

While this is a subjective scale, it has been extensively tested and shown to correlate well with objective measures such as heart rate and blood pressure. In my experience most people use the scale very effectively. However, there are two groups whom I have found don't use it correctly. The first is young, macho men, who have a sense of invincibility that only youth can confer. During a test, they may be close to collapsing with fatigue, but when shown the scale, they will rate the effort as very light (especially when the test is being conducted by a young lady). The second are frail old ladies who get so intimidated with the thought of exercise, that they rate the exertion as very hard, and that's even before they get on the treadmill!

The RPE scale can be used to prescribe exercise across activities. For example, you could exercise at an intensity which feels fairly light or somewhat hard to you, whether you are running, cycling, swimming, or even lifting weights. In my opinion the RPE scale is a great tool to monitor exercise and is not used often enough.

Rate of Perceived Exertion (RPE) Scale

6	
7	VERY, VERY LIGHT
8	
9	VERY LIGHT
10	
11	FAIRLY LIGHT
12	
13	SOMEWHAT HARD
14	
15	HARD
16	
17	VERY HARD
18	
19	VERY, VERY HARD
20	

3. Talk test

The simplest way to measure exercise intensity is the talk test.

When I was in school our PT (physical training) master would warn us not to talk during exercise (or laugh, or smile, or drink water—amongst the many rules that we had to follow). Hopefully, no one will monitor you as strictly, so when you are exercising at a moderate intensity, you should be able to talk without getting out of breath. However, if you are able to sing comfortably, then you are probably not working hard enough. On the other hand, if you are able to speak only in gasps, then you may need to slow down.

As you can see, there are a number of ways that one can measure exercise intensity, ranging from objective to subjective. Trainers will tell you that exercising at low intensity burns more fat, but exercising at high intensity burns more calories. So, which is better? I have a simple rule of thumb.

Initially do not worry about intensity; work on building up exercise time to about 45 minutes. Once you do that, work on increasing the intensity. Ultimately, you will reach a plateau where you will be able to exercise for 30 to 60 minutes at the highest intensity that you can comfortably sustain. This will usually be somewhere between 70–85 per cent of your max heart rate.

Post-script: Jaideep had an injury and has stopped long distance running, so we cycle together now. Unfortunately, he applies the same principle to cycling as well. He gets into the highest gear, literally, from the get go. Guess he hasn't read this chapter yet!

Time—Exercise duration

The amount of time you are able to exercise is related to the intensity of exercise. The ideal is to find a combination which allows you to sustain exercise at an appropriate heart rate for a reasonable amount of time. The guidelines state that doing 30 minutes of moderate intensity exercise five times a week is equivalent to doing 20 minutes of vigorous exercise three times a week. My personal advice is to aim for 30-60 minutes of continuous exercise at moderate intensity. To reach this level, you need to build up gradually and your starting point will depend on your current fitness level and health status.

What about splitting exercise into smaller parts?

In the past, all research looking at exercise studied bouts of 20 minutes or longer. It was assumed that only after 20 minutes did the health benefits of exercise kick in. However, over the last decade, it has been shown that exercise can be broken up into smaller bouts through the day, and the benefits derived are similar to those you get from a single session. Specifically, it was shown that three bouts of 10 minutes each is equivalent to a single bout of 30 minutes. This is comforting for those who are not fit or healthy enough to sustain exercise for more than 10 minutes at a time, especially older individuals and those with medical conditions such as osteoarthritis.

I often meet patients who say they are very busy and therefore 10-minute sessions sound like a great idea. Is it a great idea, or is it an excuse to get away with less? In my mind the real effort is getting the exercise session started.

Once you have started, then adding some more time is easier than adding two more short sessions during the day.

Type of exercise

The final 'T' in the exercise prescription is for the type of exercise you need to do. The simplest example of aerobic exercise is walking. It's an activity which we are all comfortable doing, and when done in an exercise format has great health benefits. However, all too often I see groups of walkers who are engrossed in conversations about the stock market, or about the latest antics of our politicians, and they are merely strolling along. There is nothing wrong in walking in groups (in fact, I encourage it), or carrying on a conversation, but often, in the process, the actual walk suffers. As was mentioned earlier, you do need to get your heart rate up in the target zone to derive maximal benefits from exercise.

Other common forms of aerobic exercise include running, cycling (both indoors and outdoors), swimming, and gym-based equipment, such as the elliptical or cross-trainer which is very popular these days.

Is walking the best exercise?

Whenever I give a talk to a large group of people, I invariably get asked the question, 'Which is the best exercise?' Often, before I can answer, someone from the audience pipes up, 'Walking, of course!' Walking is certainly a great exercise, but is it the 'best' exercise? The answer is yes and no, so let me explain.

You should start your exercise program with walking at a comfortable pace for a few minutes. Gradually build up to 30-60 minutes of walking at a brisk pace, and then maintain this for a while. However, once you have achieved this, and there are no health reasons preventing you from doing more, then it certainly is beneficial to increase the pace and even start running for short stretches. In fact, you could do a walk-run combination, with the run component getting longer as your fitness increases. The health benefits of running do exceed those of walking for the equivalent time period. But running does put an increased strain on your muscles and bones, and the risk of injury tends to be more than that for walking. Therefore you need to find a balance between increasing the intensity and your injury risk.

To get back to the original question, I think walking is the best exercise from a public health perspective, but from an individual perspective, once you have been walking regularly there is added benefit in increasing the intensity and adding running to your routine.

Warming up and cooling down

Since school days, we have been taught to warm up before undertaking exercise. In those days, a warm-up meant doing vigorous stretching exercises, and jumping up and down.

The purpose of a warm-up is to gradually get your body ready for exercise by slowly increasing your heart rate, and literally 'warming up' your muscles, which is done by increasing their blood flow. For that purpose, the simplest and best warm-up would be to start with your intended exercise, but to do it at a much lighter pace for the first five minutes. So, whether it's swimming, walking, or cycling, you can start the activity at a much slower pace initially and gradually build it up.

While most of us take this advice seriously, we don't do such a good job when it comes to cooling down at the end of exercise (and I must confess that I am guilty of this myself). Ideally, the last few minutes of exercise should be done at a reduced pace before coming to a complete stop. This is especially true of activities like running and brisk walking. When you suddenly stop after a long run, blood tends to 'pool' in your legs and you end up feeling light-headed and may even fall over.

Where should you exercise?

Broadly speaking, you can exercise indoors or outdoors, and the decision of where is a matter of personal choice. As the saying goes, one man's food is another man's poison; similarly, the benefits of the outdoors for some may be viewed as negatives by others. The outdoors allows you to breathe in fresh air, but at the same time you breathe in the pollution too. Some will view the outdoor weather conditions as a plus, while others will prefer the controlled temperature of the indoors. Some will cite the attraction of television viewing indoors as an advantage, while others will argue that the entertainment on our city streets is far superior to any saas-bahu serial. When exercising outdoors, you need to keep a watchful eye on traffic. Cycling in a city like Mumbai is far more dangerous than any *Khatron ke Khiladi* reality TV episode.

Walking on the treadmill

There is one myth I would like to explode at this point, and that's related to walking on the treadmill. Somehow, it's cemented in people's minds that walking outdoors is fine, but walking on a treadmill will land you in all sorts of trouble for your knees and joints. There is no scientific truth in that. Walking is a weight-bearing exercise with impact (unlike cycling for example), and consequently puts a certain amount of stress on your joints. However, the stress is not more if you walk on a treadmill. In fact, you could justifiably argue that the treadmill is a smooth and cushioned surface unlike the roads in most of our cities, and hence may even be a safer option from an injury perspective.

What time of day should you exercise?

There is a deep-seated belief in most people that a morning walk is the best form of exercise. In fact it's often used in conversation as one word—morning walk—and most consider it strange to exercise at any other time. Actually, there is no specific best time of the day to exercise. You can derive the benefits of exercise at any time of day. However, you should not exercise for about two hours after a meal, though there can be considerable variation in this rule, depending on how large your meal was and how strenuous is the planned exercise.

The reason for not exercising after a meal is quite simple. You need extra blood flow to the stomach and other digestive organs after eating, and you need extra blood flow to muscles while exercising (the demand can go up by more than 10-fold). So, if you exercise immediately after eating then there is a tug-of-war for blood flow between the stomach and the muscles, which is why you may experience discomfort in your abdomen.

In summary, the best type of exercise, the best location of exercise and the best time of day to exercise, is what you consider most enjoyable and will stick with for a long time, hopefully forever. People often get lost in the fine details of exercise and end up making complicated programs, which they cannot adhere to. I would rather you start with a simple plan which fits in well with your lifestyle and then scale it up, once you taste initial success.

Strength training

Mrs Urmila Vasudev was 72 years old and had started cardiac rehabilitation after her bypass surgery. After a few weeks, I told her in the presence of her family that she was ready to begin some strength training. They all looked at me strangely for suggesting that a 72-year-old lady who has had a heart attack and bypass surgery should be lifting weights.

I have had this reaction before, and almost expect it every time I talk about strength training, also called weight or resistance training. When most people hear the term 'strength training', they think of Salman Khan wearing a tight sleeveless vest with his muscles rippling, and simply cannot see how we could recommend it for heart patients. However, if I had to ask the same lady to lift a bottle of water at home for 10 repetitions once a day, it would not seem so strange. Lifting a one litre bottle of water is the same as lifting a one kg weight and would qualify as strength training. Lifting very heavy weights for the purpose of bodybuilding is different from light training to maintain good health.

For several decades weight training was considered taboo for anyone with heart disease. The fear was that lifting weights would cause a sharp spike in blood pressure, which could be dangerous. However, research done over the past two decades has shown that strength training is not only safe, but is also extremely beneficial for all, including those with heart disease. Most of the benefits that we get with cardio training, such as an improved lipid profile, better sugar, BP, and weight control, can also be seen with strength training. In addition, it helps increase your muscle mass and reduce body fat, which increases metabolism and aids in weight loss. Today, the guidelines state that after a few weeks of a cardiac event, patients can safely participate and benefit from a strength-training program.

Strength-training program

The FITT principle can also be applied to strength training:

- F – Frequency – two or three days a week is adequate to get health benefits from strength training
- I – Intensity – we usually do not use heart rate guidelines for strength training, and it would be better to use the RPE scale, on which your exertion level should be between 11–13 (fairly light to somewhat hard).
- T – Time. There is no fixed duration that is recommended for a strength training session, but usually a session should last between 20–45 minutes.
- T – Type. Strength training includes lifting weights, as well as using your body weight as resistance, or using elastic resistance bands. It is usually described in sets and repetitions. For example, if you are exercising your biceps (upper arm), each time you lift the weight up is called one repetition and a continuous set of repetitions (also called 'reps') make up one set. Ideally, each set should consist of 10–15 reps. Circuit training is a type of weight training in which you do a number of exercises and move from one exercise to another, with about half a minute's gap between each exercise. This tends to keep your heart rate elevated, and you also get a bit of an aerobic or cardio workout.

How should you get started?

Most of us have probably not done any form of weight training in our lives, so it's important to get started at a low level and then gradually build up. It's a good idea to start initially with resistance bands, which are colour-coded for different resistance levels. If you do not want to buy special equipment, you could even use household items to provide the weight. My late grandmother was 80 years old when I first encouraged her to lift weights, and we started with a half litre bottle of water, with which she did different exercises for her arms and shoulders (and looked mighty cute while doing it, I might add).

At this point you may wonder why older individuals should lift weights, and the answer is quite simple. As we age, we begin to lose muscle mass, and as that happens, our activities of daily living get affected too. Even simple

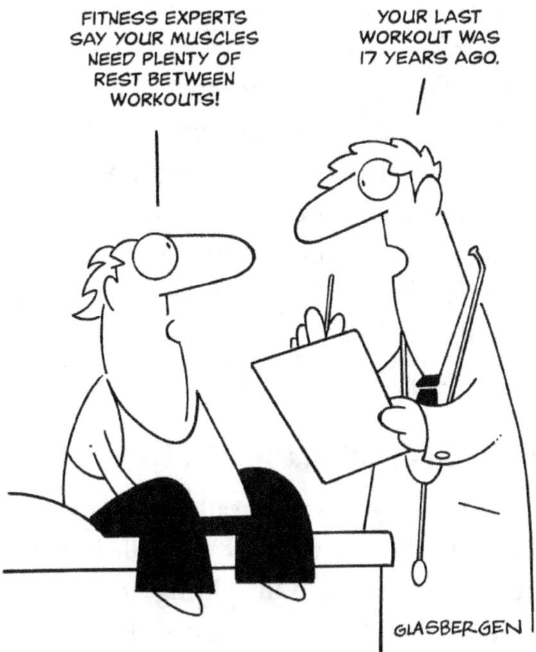

©Randy Glasbergen   www.glasbergen.com

household activities, such as lifting a bag of groceries or moving a bucket, require strength, and the more active muscle mass we have, the easier it is to perform these activities. One of the biggest pitfalls in old age is having a fall and subsequent fracture. Regular exercise, including weight training, has been shown to strengthen the muscles and bones, and greatly reduce the risk of falls and fractures.

Once you are comfortable with resistance bands, you can progress to light hand weights (dumbbells) and machines. The advantage of using free weights is that they allow a greater range of motion, which can be a problem if the form is wrong. On the other hand, machines restrict your movement in a particular range, which is preferred if you are lifting heavy weights.

In the initial few months, you should be doing 8-10 exercises, which can be divided into the upper and lower body. You should do one set of each exercise, and each set should consist of 10-15 reps. As you progress and get comfortable with this routine, you can increase the number of sets you do per exercise and also increase the number of exercises. Research has shown that for general health benefits even one set per exercise is good enough, but if you enjoy it and want greater gains, you can progress to three sets per exercise.

There is an easy rule of thumb when deciding how much weight to lift. Select a weight that allows you to complete 10-15 reps of the exercise comfortably. If the weight is so light that you can easily do more than 20 reps, then you need to increase it, and if it's so heavy that you can barely complete 8 reps, then you need to reduce it. Start with a light weight, but over time, it's important to gradually increase the weight, for sustained benefits.

Precautions while lifting weights

It's important to pay attention to your breathing while weight training. Most people tend to instinctively hold their breath while lifting weights, and this leads to a rise in blood pressure. While lifting, it's important to maintain a normal breathing pattern. It's recommended that you breathe out when you lift the weight (effort phase) and breathe in when you lower the weight.

If you have had bypass surgery you should wait for at least six weeks before lifting weights overhead, or any exercise putting a strain on your chest region. This is the amount of time it takes the breast bone to heal after open heart surgery.

It is also important to focus on your form while doing strength exercises. Many people have a habit of doing them in a hurry and use momentum to lift the weight, which will deprive you of the complete benefit of a strength workout, besides increasing your risk for injury.

Exercise guidelines for cardiovascular and strength training

	CARDIOVASCULAR EXERCISE	STRENGTH TRAINING	COMMENTS
Frequency	Daily for moderate intensity exercise. 3-5 days per week for high intensity	2-3 days per week	Aim to decrease 'sedentary' time as much as possible
Intensity	60-85 per cent of max HR, or 11-13 on RPE scale	11-13 on RPE scale	Listen to your body. Slow down and stop if you get symptoms, such as chest discomfort or shortness of breath
Time	30-60 minutes	Complete one set of 8-10 exercises. Each set should be 10-15 reps	Can be broken down into smaller bouts of 10 min each
Type	Walking, running, cycling, swimming, cardio gym equipment	Resistance bands, dumbbells, weight machines	The 'best' exercise is the one you enjoy the most

Exercise for those with heart disease

The first time I met Sam Balsara, he was in a wheelchair. Sam is one of the giants of the Indian advertising world, and is the founder and Chairman of Madison World, the largest independent advertising firm in the country. He had just had bypass surgery two months ago, and had a prolonged hospital stay. I expected to meet a gregarious outgoing marketing personality, but the surgery had taken a toll on him, mentally and physically. He was on a wheelchair, since he got out of breath at the slightest exertion. I assured him and his family that we would get him better than before, very soon, and they looked hopeful, though a bit sceptical.

The first time he exercised in cardiac rehab he walked just a few steps and was out of breath. Actually, this is not unusual. Many patients after a heart attack or surgery are extremely deconditioned. This is a combination of the actual heart ailment as well as the prolonged bed rest that often accompanies it. In addition, the disease tends to have a huge psychological burden, which tends to have physical manifestations. I am happy to tell you that we were able to progress Mr Balsara quite rapidly after the initial few weeks, and he achieved full recovery. Now, it's great to see him every Saturday at cardiac rehab, in spite of his busy schedule, looking quite dapper in his Delhi Marathon tracksuit, exercising for over an hour at a high level. I had the pleasure of attending the 25th anniversary party of Madison World, and Sam was the star of the evening. He was a very far cry from the man I saw huddled on a wheelchair a year ago.

Build it up gradually

The principles of exercise do not change if you have heart disease; however, there are certain precautions you need to take to ensure safety.

As discussed in the earlier part of the chapter, the goal is to achieve 30-60 minutes of exercise per day, but that does not mean you need to achieve it on day one. In fact, that would be the wrong thing to do. After you have been discharged from the hospital, start with walking for 5 to 10 minutes, 4 times a day. Each week, increase the time by 5 to 10 minutes. When you are able to walk 20 minutes at a stretch, you can reduce the frequency to twice a day, and when you reach 30-60 minutes, once a day is good enough. After a heart attack or bypass surgery, it should take you about six weeks to reach this goal. The process could be shortened by a couple of weeks if you have had an elective angioplasty (as opposed to an emergency one). For a detailed week-by-week program, please refer to the chapters on bypass surgery and angioplasty. Each patient is different, and some may need to take greater precaution, especially those who have an ejection fraction of less than 35 per cent. However, a low ejection fraction does not mean that you cannot achieve your goals; it may just take you a couple of weeks longer to do so.

Special precautions

While exercising you need to be particularly aware of any symptoms such as angina or shortness of breath. If you recollect, in an earlier chapter we had discussed angina, and the important message was that it did not always manifest as pain on the left side of the chest. In fact, in most instances it presents itself in some other form, and it's important to remember that any discomfort in the upper part of the body, from navel to nose, which increases with exertion, should be viewed as angina, unless proven otherwise. I had a patient whose angina manifested as an aching in the jaw and teeth every time he walked fast. That was his 'anginal equivalent', and it has been documented in most people that their anginal equivalent usually remains the same over time. If you do notice angina, unusual shortness of breath or fatigue with exercise, then you need to stop exercising and seek the advice of your doctor before continuing with exercise. We have all heard the phrase 'no pain, no gain', but this is absolutely not true when it comes to heart disease and exercise. It's fine to push yourself a little if your leg muscles are aching a bit, but if you have chest discomfort, you need to stop immediately.

Unusual shortness of breath and sweating

It's worth taking a moment at this point to explain the concept of unusual shortness of breath or fatigue.

Let's say a person lives on the fourth floor of a building without an elevator and has gotten used to climbing the stairs over the last 10 years, and can do it comfortably. If this person now gets out of breath within three floors, then he is experiencing unusual shortness of breath with usual activity, and needs to consult his doctor. On the other hand, you have a person who always takes the elevator, and on the rare occasion when he needs to climb three flights of steps, he is out of breath. This person does not need to see his doctor, but rather needs to see a fitness instructor.

When you exercise outdoors, especially in our weather conditions, it's normal to sweat. This is a mechanism by which the body releases excess heat, and is much needed. If the sweating is excessive for the activity undertaken, then it might be of concern, but what is excessive is also dependent on the weather conditions. It's normal to sweat a lot when walking outdoors in summer even for a short distance. On the other hand, if you sweat while taking a short walk in an air-conditioned room, that may need to be investigated.

Exercise for diabetics

There are two types of diabetes, Type 1 and Type 2. In Type 1, the body does not make insulin, which is the hormone required to regulate blood sugar. People suffering from Type 1 diabetes need to take insulin shots their entire life. Type 2 diabetes usually develops later in life and is more related to lifestyle, and is also known as adult onset diabetes. These diabetics usually have enough insulin, but suffer from 'insulin resistance', in which the muscles are not adequately able to use the insulin to regulate blood sugar. In either case, exercise has a tremendous benefit and has an insulin-like effect. In all my years of practice, I have come across more than 25,000 readings of patients' blood sugars before and after exercise. It's amazing to see how effectively a simple bout of moderate intensity exercise can control blood sugar. It's not uncommon to see a 100-150 point drop in sugar before and after exercise. The human body has this great ability to normalize blood sugar with exercise. So, if a patient's sugar is 240 mg/dl before exercise, it might drop to 120 mg/dl after exercise. However, if the same person starts exercise the next day with a sugar of 180 mg/dl, it may drop to 130 mg/dl.

For diabetics, it's important to have a balance between food intake, exercise and medication to normalize sugar readings, and certain special precautions need to be taken.

Special considerations for diabetics

Exercise reduces blood sugar, which is great, but sometimes it's possible that medication and exercise combined may reduce sugar to a hypoglycaemic level. So it's important to monitor blood glucose (with a glucometer) before and after exercise, at least for the first few times. Signs of hypoglycaemia (low blood sugar) include sweating, light-headedness, nausea, and a general feeling of uneasiness. Unfortunately, signs of hyperglycaemia (high blood sugar) are also very similar. When in doubt, measure the sugar, and if you are not able to do that, it's safer to assume that the signs are due to low blood sugar, and give the person sugar, rather than assume it to be high and withhold sugar.

The insulin dose and site of injection may need to be adjusted when you start exercising. It is preferable to inject insulin in the stomach area rather than legs before exercise. Most exercises use your leg muscles, and during exercise these muscles absorb insulin very quickly, which could lead to a sudden fall in sugar (coupled with the fall which exercise will cause, in any case).

Examine your feet for any injury on a regular basis. Some diabetics lose sensation in their feet and may not feel minor injuries, which then increase and cause complications like ulcers.

Avoid starting exercise if your blood sugar is more than 300 mg/dl. Meet with your doctor and get the sugar under better control first.

Always keep a 'sugar snack' by your side while exercising. I suggest you keep a sachet of sugar in your pocket, especially if you are on insulin, since there is a higher chance of hypoglycaemia occurring post exercise for those on insulin. This sachet can be consumed if you feel signs and symptoms of hypoglycaemia such as light-headedness. Earlier I used to suggest keeping a piece of chocolate but then I found out very quickly that most patients got tempted and ate the chocolate even when their sugar was normal!

Make sure you wear a good pair of walking shoes with adequate cushioning to protect your feet. It is equally important to change your shoes on a regular basis, such as after every 500-700 kilometres of walking. Of late there has been a new fad towards running barefoot, or running in shoes with a very thin sole (like the white canvas shoes we wore in school). However, I would not advise this for diabetics, especially outdoors, as the risk for surface injuries would greatly increase.

Safety of exercise

Ranjan Das was 42 years old and the CEO of the multinational information technology company SAP in India. After exercising one morning he returned to his apartment and had a massive heart attack and unfortunately died soon after (may God rest his soul). This tragedy made headlines and once again the question was raised on the safety of exercise.

The truth is that a very miniscule amount of people die during exercise, while a thousand times more have an attack just lying down in bed or sitting on the sofa and watching TV at home. Yet, how many times have you read a headline saying 'Man has heart attack while watching TV at home'. Ironically, the only time that headline does happen is if the person was watching a critical cricket or football game in which his favourite team was playing and lost the match. In these cases, someone else exercising caused their heart attack!

While you are exercising, your physiological parameters are on the higher side, and for that brief period your risk is more than while you are at rest. Your risk at rest can be considered your baseline risk, which drops considerably over time with regular exercise. This is a bit complicated so allow me to illustrate by using an example. Let's assume that you are a sedentary person and your risk of having an attack is 8 per cent throughout the day. When you exercise that risk may go up a bit to say, 9 per cent. (Please note these numbers are not real figures; they're being used only to explain the point.) Now, if you start a regular exercise program, your baseline risk might drop to 5 per cent throughout the day, but for the brief period you exercise, it might rise to 6 per cent. If you do not follow this closely do not worry, all you need to remember is that with regular exercise your risk for heart attack and death drops significantly.

In a large study looking at long-distance running over the past decade in the US, it was found that out of 11 million runners who participated there were only 42 deaths in all those years. To put it in perspective, this amounts to a death rate of 0.0002 per cent per year, while the death rate from a car accident is 100 times higher.

While exercise is an extremely safe activity for all, including those with heart disease, it is important to follow appropriate precautions while exercising.

Is there something like too much exercise?

One morning at work, Mrs Asha Puri pulled me aside and said she wanted to have a word. Her husband Chetan had undergone an angioplasty four months ago, and was following up regularly in cardiac rehab. To give him moral support and to take care of herself, she had enrolled in our preventive program, though she was extremely fit. I was wondering what was up, when she told me in a worried tone, 'Doc, I think Chetan is overdoing it. He is exercising in rehab three days a week, is playing golf three days a week and lifts weights too. I am worried that this may be too much for his heart, please talk to him.' My reply surprised her, when I said, 'That's great, more power to him. He's really taking care of himself.' I don't know whether she was reassured, but she seemed to accept my answer grudgingly.

Of course, it did get me thinking if there was something like too much exercise. Studies have found that the best benefit of exercise is obtained when you burn between 700 to 3,500 calories per week. After that there is no further benefit, and some have even shown negative effects of exercising more than 3,500 calories per week. But don't get worried about over-exercising so soon, since it's not easy to burn that many calories. Walking or running one mile (1.6 km) burns approximately 100 calories. So, to burn 3500, you would need to walk/run for 35 miles (55 km) a week, which is not that easy to do.

Beware the weekend warrior!

The other day at the hospital, I was speaking with Dr Akshay Mehta, a cardiologist and sportsman himself. He was narrating to me an incident of someone who died on the badminton court at his local gymkhana. Apparently the person had not been active for several years and then one day came out and played a strenuous game for hours.

Sudden, unaccustomed exercise is dangerous for your heart and needs to be avoided. If you are beginning an exercise program or are getting back to exercise after a long gap, make sure you start very slowly and progress gradually. Most people have not been active since their college days and then want to get back to their former levels of fitness in a hurry. You can always recover your lost glory, but make sure you take your time in getting there.

Dealing with injuries

If you exercise regularly, you may come across minor aches and pains in your muscles and joints. For most of these injuries, the simplest form of treatment can be summarized by the acronym RICE, which stands for rest, ice, compression and elevation.

Most injuries are due to some form of inflammatory process occurring, and ice is the best treatment for acute injuries. I prefer real ice being used, instead of an ice pack, and the best way to apply it is to fill a polythene bag with a dozen cubes of ice and rest it on the injured part for 10-15 minutes. At first it will be hard to bear the cold and the tendency will be to remove it every couple of minutes, but after a while you should be able to leave it on for the necessary time. Try and do this two to three times a day, especially if the pain persists. If you don't feel better soon, or if the injury is serious to begin with, then you should consult with a physiotherapist or an orthopaedic doctor right away.

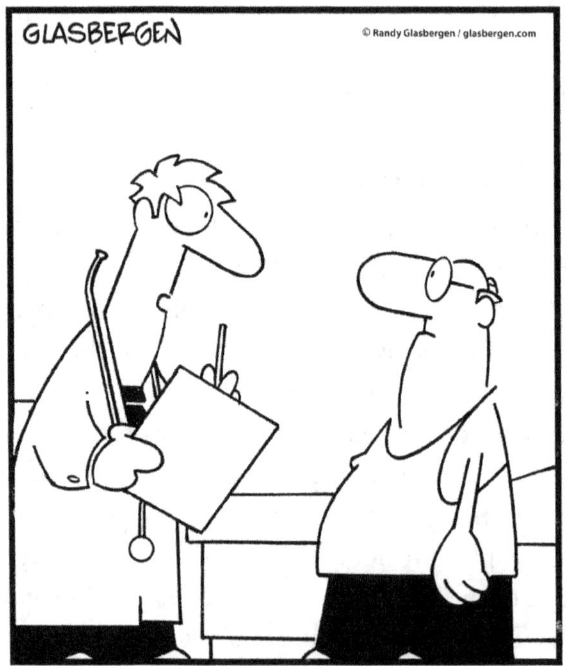

"What fits your busy schedule better, exercising one hour a day or being dead 24 hours a day?"

Excuses to avoid exercise

Mrs Chandaben Mehta was a 58-year-old homemaker who met me for a consult. Her triglycerides were 207 mg/dl, her fasting blood sugar was 124 mg/dl, and she was about 10 kilos overweight. I told her that the good news was that she did not need to start medication right away, but ought to make lifestyle changes, which included a daily walk for 45 minutes. Without batting an eyelid, she told me that she agreed with me, but she just did not have the time to exercise. This amused me, and I asked her how it was that she did not have one hour out of 24 for exercise?

She then proceeded to chalk out her day, which started with a visit to the Derasar, followed by giving her domestic help instructions, followed by giving her husband his medications, followed by lunch and a short nap (she just 'lies down', but does not sleep, to quote her accurately). In the evening, she had to shop at the bazaar, organize dinner for the family, and then arrange for her son's tiffin the next day (her daughter-in-law was not capable of this, according to her).

As you can tell from the above narrative, it's not that Mrs Shah does not have time to exercise; it's just that exercise is not her priority. This whole concept of not having time in my opinion is the greatest false excuse in the world for not exercising. Let me ask you this—have you brushed your teeth this morning, or had a bath? The answer is clearly yes. I recommend my patients to treat exercise as part of their daily routine, on the same level as eating, bathing, and sleeping. Somehow we always manage these, irrespective of whatever else we are doing, since we consider them as essential parts of our daily routine. Similarly, we need to start looking at exercise as a normal part of our day and not 'something extra' we end up doing.

Another very common reason given, especially by executives, is that they are travelling all the time. My usual response to that excuse is, 'I assume there is a road in the place you are travelling to, and if there is no road, then it's even better for your knees to walk on a natural surface.' Of course, I say that in jest, but the point is that often it's not a lack of will to exercise, but a lack of creativity in knowing how to fit exercise into your schedule. In fact, travel is one of the best situations to exercise. You end up sitting for hours in airport lounges, during which time you could walk up and down in the terminal and get in your extra steps (and maybe some strange looks) in the process. Also, when you travel, there is usually no family or social commitments and you have more time on hand after the day's business is over.

'Real reasons' to avoid exercise

Besides all the precautions we have spoken about, you need to listen to your body when it sends you signals. Do not exercise when you are unwell, or are generally feeling below the weather. Often regular exercisers get addicted to the high of exercise and ignore these warnings, which sometimes lead to dangerous consequences. Rest and recovery are essential parts of your training, and should not be compromised.

Avoid strenuous activity, when you have not had adequate sleep, especially after long journeys.

Over a period of time if you find that you are getting fatigued quicker than usual, you need to pay attention to that. If may be a consequence of overtraining, or it may be an early warning sign of trouble, and you should talk to your doctor.

A fit person is not a freak

Let me end the exercise section by talking about one of my pet peeves. I hate it when people use the term 'fitness freak' to describe someone who exercises regularly and makes it a part of his or her life. I know it's meant to be complimentary, but the term freak suggests something abnormal. As a society, we have become so sedentary that it's 'normal' to be inactive and 'freaky' to be exercising. Should it not be the other way around? Should we not call a lazy person a freak, and apply the label of 'star' to someone who exercises? Well, it's food for thought as you turn to the next chapter on nutrition.

Take-home messages

- Exercise is very effective in the prevention and treatment of heart disease.

- Moderate intensity exercise such as brisk walking is recommended most days of the week. Apply the FITT (frequency, intensity, time and type) guidelines to formulate your exercise prescription.

- In addition to structured exercise, it's crucial to be physically active through the day. Use a pedometer and aim to get in 10,000 steps every day.

- Strength training should be included in your plan, since it provides a range of benefits complementary to aerobic or cardiovascular training.

- The principles of exercise do not differ for those with heart disease, but care must be taken to start slow and progress gradually.

- Diabetics need to monitor their sugar before and after exercise. They may need to adjust their medication, since exercise has an insulin-like effect.

11

Nutrition

(The way to the heart is through the stomach)

ONE-QUARTER OF WHAT YOU EAT KEEPS YOU ALIVE. THE OTHER THREE-QUARTERS keeps your doctor alive. – Hieroglyph found in an ancient Egyptian tomb, 3000 BC.

Let food be thy medicine, and let thy medicine be food. – Hippocrates (father of medicine), 5th century BC.

The doctor of the future will no longer treat the human frame with drugs, but rather will cure and prevent disease with nutrition. – Thomas Edison, 20th century AD.

As you can tell from the above quotations, from 3000 BC onwards, people have recognized the relationship between food and health. No area of lifestyle modification attracts as much attention as food. Probably no area of life attracts as much attention as food. Across cultures and continents, food occupies a central place in daily life. Besides the obvious need for nourishment, it has tremendous cultural significance too. As we age, we may lose our sight and hearing, but our taste buds remain active forever.

While it is universally accepted that the food we eat has a direct bearing on our health, there are huge controversies on what constitutes a healthful diet. There are as many schools of thought on an appropriate diet as there are different cuisines in the world. Take for example the old saying, 'An apple a day keeps the doctor away.' An apple is considered by most as a symbol of good health, but if you look at some of the popular low-carbohydrate diets, an apple is something to stay away from rather than the doctor! Often, trying to keep up with the latest information on nutrition can get you more confused rather than enlightened. Also, as we are discovering more about genetics, we are learning that there are huge variations in how people react to different foods. For example, there are some cholesterol conditions which do better on a slightly higher fat diet than others. Personalized medicine, which includes personalized nutrition, is the future of medicine. Which is why I do not prescribe a one-size diet for all. I would rather educate you on various principles of heart-healthy nutrition, and give you the flexibility as well as responsibility to plan a diet to suit your needs.

The fundamentals of nutrition

Before we go into the specifics of what to eat, it's important to understand the fundamentals of nutrition. The major food groups, which constitute the largest part of our diet and provide us with energy, are carbohydrates, fats and proteins. In addition, vitamins and minerals, which we consume in smaller quantities, help in the optimal functioning of the body.

Carbohydrates

If you took a group of people from anywhere in the world without preconceived notions of dietary principles and laid out a large spread of food in front of them, their natural choice would be to consume carbohydrates (or 'carbs' as they are popularly known), in the largest quantity, followed by fat and proteins. Carbohydrates form the bulk of our food consumption and have done so for generations. It's only of late that they have gotten a bad name, and it's almost fashionable to say, 'I am off carbs,' or 'I don't eat carbs at night.'

Carbohydrates serve as the main source of energy, and each gram provides four calories (also known as kilocalories) of energy. They can broadly be divided into simple and complex. Simple carbohydrates, also known as sugars, help in providing instant energy. Sweets, cold drinks, and honey are examples of simple sugars. Complex carbs, on the other hand, take longer to digest, since they first need to be broken into simple sugars before the body absorbs them. Whole grains such as bajra, jowar and oats are examples of complex carbs and are an extremely vital and healthful part of a nutritious diet.

Fats

Fats have evoked much controversy over the last few decades, with some diet gurus advocating you to stay away from them, while others actually suggest that you eat fat to burn fat.

Fats are more calorie dense than carbs, and provide 9 calories (cals) of energy per gram. Depending on the chemical structure, fats can be divided into saturated and unsaturated. Saturated fats are usually solid at room temperature (think ghee and butter), while unsaturated fats are liquid at room temperature (think oils), and can be divided further into monounsaturated (MUFA) and polyunsaturated fatty acids (PUFA).

Fats are a great source of energy for the body, and are also essential for absorbing and utilizing vitamins A, D, E, and K (the fat soluble vitamins). Another type of fat that has come into prominence lately (for all the wrong reasons) is trans-fat. This fat is obtained by the process of partial hydrogenation of vegetable oils (think 'dalda' or 'vanaspati'), and is typically found in commercial baked goods such as cookies and pastries.

Proteins

Proteins are the building blocks of our body. They are required for the structure and function of various organs in the body. They also help speed up several of the biochemical reactions needed for life.

Proteins are made up of links of different amino acids. There are about 20 different amino acids, of which 8 are known as essential amino acids since they cannot be made by the body, and need to be obtained directly through diet. The other 12 can be synthesized within the body.

Proteins are not primarily used as a source of energy, but like carbs, they give 4 calories of energy per gram. Indian diets are often deficient in proteins, though it's a misconception that adequate protein cannot be consumed through a vegetarian diet. Milk, paneer, beans and legumes are good examples of vegetarian protein. The daily protein requirement for most people is 0.8 gm/kg body weight and can be obtained through healthy eating.

Diet for heart patients

Rusi Vimadalal had his angioplasty at the age of 60, and met me with his wife about two weeks after the event. He looked thoroughly depressed, which is not uncommon for those who have recently suffered. I tried to reassure him by telling him that the worst was over, and now he would be able to lead a full and healthy life. That's when he blurted out, 'Doctor, it's the future I am worried about. My wife is forcing me to eat all this ghaas-foos; how can I survive on it? And that too, it's all boiled! How is it possible for me to look forward to a life of this torture?'

Rusi was a lifelong non-vegetarian, and grew up looking at vegetables as the enemy. After his heart attack, everyone around him had told him that he needed to immediately turn vegetarian. Those of you who know Parsis well will know that a 'vegetarian Parsi' is a contradiction in terms, though a few of them do exist. There is a month in the Parsi calendar where believers are enjoined to be vegetarian, but even during that month fish and eggs are fair play! So, it's not so hard to understand the plight of poor Rusi. When I told him that he did not have to be a total vegetarian, the smile came back to his face, and I became his new best friend.

The diet that needs to be followed by heart patients is actually not very different from so-called normal people. I say 'so-called normal' since many have underlying health issues such as diabetes, hypertension, and even heart disease, which they are unaware of.

When I am counselling patients on diet, it is usual to have their family members sitting with them. The patient usually has a glum look on his face, since he expects me to add insult to his myocardial injury by giving a long list of things he can never eat. Meanwhile, the family members are looking on, with a look which seems to suggest, 'We have told you to stop eating all the "good" things; now hear it directly from the doctor's mouth.' In such situations it gives me great pleasure to inform them that the patient's food should not be cooked separately. The food that the patient is eating is actually what should be consumed by *all* family members. This is where a reversal of looks takes place, and the patient finally smiles (with a look that suggests, 'If I am going to suffer, I am happy you are going to suffer too'), while it's the turn of the family members to turn glum. I point out that cooking separately is like saying that the entire family should eat in an unhealthy manner until they suffer from heart disease! Before *you* begin to turn glum, let me reassure you that the diet I am about to prescribe has many foods that you can eat, and very few that you should restrict.

What's the right mix of food groups?

The bulk of studies looking at heart disease have shown that consuming a diet which is low in fat and high in complex carbohydrates reduces cardiac risk factors, as well as heart attacks and deaths. However, over the last decade, there has been renewed interest in low carbohydrate regimens, with a special focus on their ability to cause weight loss. The most popular of the low carb diets is the Atkins diet, in which carbohydrate intake is about 5-10 per cent, proteins are 25-30 per cent, and fats make up the rest. There are several variations of this diet, all of which keep the carb intake at less than 40 per cent. At the other extreme are the very low-fat diets, the most popular of which is the Ornish diet, in which total fat is kept to less than 10 per cent and carbs are as high as 75 per cent.

The scientific community had shunned the very low-carb diets for years, but due to their growing popularity among dieters, a number of studies in which carb intake is severely restricted have now been carried out and their findings present an interesting picture. In head-to-head studies of low- versus high-carb diets, the former caused greater initial weight loss at six months, but when followed for a year or longer, the weight loss evened out. One of the concerns of low-carb diets was their effect on cholesterol and sugar, but surprisingly in the short-term, these parameters improved for the better. Most of this improvement could be attributed to weight loss achieved through the diet. In studies, it has been seen that as long as there is weight loss, the cardiac risk parameters will improve, irrespective of the exact diet content. Having said that, the long-term (more than two years) safety and efficacy of low-carbohydrate diets have not been established, while those of a low-fat diet have.

One of the key factors for long-term success is your adherence to the diet plan. People tend to pick and choose aspects of different plans to suit their convenience, and find that they are not getting results. Imagine if you decided to eat fats as recommended by the Atkins plan, and carbs as recommended by the Ornish plan! You would end up gaining a lot of weight and your metabolic parameters would go haywire. My personal philosophy is to design a plan that you are able to sustain over a lifetime, even if that means making minor compromises. I have always maintained that a less-than perfect diet which the patient sticks to is better than a perfect diet which the patient does not follow.

After having read the research extensively, I would suggest a diet with the following break-up of the major food groups. Keep in mind that within these numbers there can be a lot of variation, and the 'quality' of carbs, fat and protein consumed has as much bearing as the total quantity consumed. This is also the reason why I have suggested a range for each of these macronutrients, and not given fixed numbers.

Nutrient	Percentage of total calories	Comment
Carbohydrates	50-60 per cent	Majority from complex carbs
Fat	20-30 per cent	Saturated fat less than 10 per cent
Protein	15-20 per cent	Tends to be low in the average Indian diet

Dietary principles

This book hopes to address a wide variety of people belonging to different ethnic groups from different parts of the country and the world. While we are all human beings, culturally we eat very differently, and there is no single approach to food that can justifiably claim to be the best. When I consult with an individual patient, I suggest a very personalized diet, but that's after I understand the patient, medically, physically and mentally.

To keep it simple, I recommend five guiding principles of diet. Under each of these principles I hope to touch upon all relevant aspects of heart-healthy nutrition. I am sure you have a million questions related to food, and all of them will not be answered in one chapter, but I do hope to equip you with enough information to plan a healthful diet for yourself.

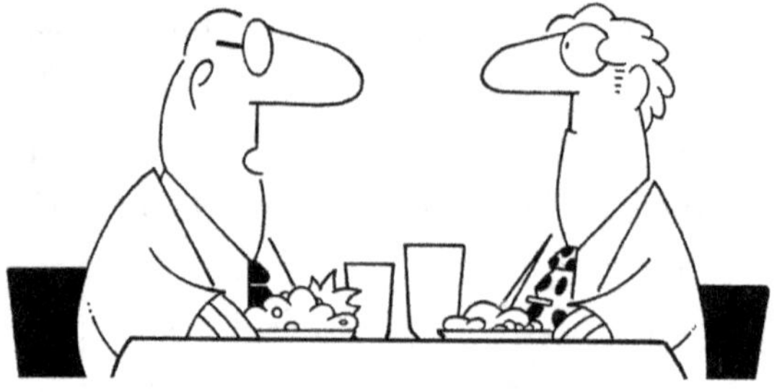

"The 4 basic food groups are things my doctor won't let me eat, things my wife won't let me eat, things my heartburn won't let me eat and things my teeth won't let me eat."

The five dietary principles

1. 1:2:3 of diet—eat from all food groups
2. Focus on fruits and vegetables
3. Make it complex
4. Keep an eye on fat intake
5. Size matters—portion size and weight control

Principle No. 1

1:2:3 of diet—Eat from all food groups

Imagine going to a restaurant and, when the waiter comes for your order, you ask for a large plate of complex carbohydrates, along with a medium serving of proteins and fats, garnished with a dash of simple sugars, and a side order of fibre. The poor chap is going to be thoroughly confused, and won't know what to bring you. Similarly, when we break up our daily intake into percentages of food groups, it makes scientific sense, but becomes difficult to implement.

When we eat food, we eat it as a whole, and don't look at it purely as carbohydrate, fat or protein. Most foods that we eat will contain a mix of these nutrients in varying proportions. The traditional Indian way of eating food is in a thali, and the food is served in small bowls, commonly called vatis or katoris, which are placed within the thali. The ingredients of the thali are usually salad, vegetables, dal, rice and rotis. My Gujarati friends call it RDBS—roti, dal, bhaat, shaak (subzi). To make it easier to understand and implement, think of six vatis or portions in your thali for every meal you eat. The principles will remain the same even when you are eating meals which do not strictly fit into the thali concept, for example when you are eating Continental or Chinese food. Divide your plate into six equal portions, and fill it using the 1:2:3 rule.

Have one portion of protein

Proteins are an important component of your diet and are often lacking in the traditional Indian diet. It's a misconception that vegetarians cannot get sufficient protein. There are several rich sources of protein in the Indian vegetarian diet. Pulses and beans such as chole, rajma, chana and green grams are an excellent source of proteins. Lentils (dals), which are a staple of our diet, contain plenty of protein, as do vegetables like green peas and spinach. Nuts like almonds and walnuts are also a great protein source, with wonderful health properties when eaten in moderation. Besides these, milk and milk products such as yogurt and paneer are also rich in protein. One portion is the amount which fits in one vati, and is approximately 100 calories. If you are non-vegetarian, you may have one serving of chicken or fish instead. One serving of chicken or fish is the size of a deck of cards. Consume red meat such as mutton and lamb sparingly.

In addition, make sure that your two portions of grains, and three of vegetables are also good protein sources. The daily protein requirement is 0.8 gm per kilogram body weight. So, a person weighing 70 kg would need 56 gm of protein a day. This can be broken down roughly into 15–20 gm protein for lunch and dinner, and the rest through breakfast and snacks.

Have two portions of grains

Rice or rotis are the preferred choice of grains in our diet. Unpolished or brown rice is healthier than white rice, and rotis made from whole-wheat atta, bajra, and jowar are much better choices than those made from flour (maida). One portion is the equivalent of one vati of rice or two small rotis. It is also okay to mix and match, where you can have one vati of rice and two small rotis.

Have three portions of vegetables

One portion is the equivalent of one vati. Vegetables should form the mainstay of your diet, and it's important to include a wide variety. The more colourful, the better. It's a good idea to select vegetables which have higher protein content. If you have not included dal in your protein portion, you could include it here. The thicker the dal, the higher the protein content.

In addition to the above, it's a great idea to start your meal with a salad of green leafy vegetables. As I had mentioned earlier, foods are never 'only' carbs or fats or proteins. So, in your protein portion, you will get some carbs, and in your vegetable and grains portion, you will get some proteins. Some amount of fat will be present in most of these items as well as your cooking medium, so fats don't need to be consumed separately. The above meal should give you roughly 600 calories, which is appropriate for most individuals consuming a 2,000 calorie per day diet. Your individual nutritional requirements may be higher, but keep the proportions of food groups the same. This will allow you to get the right mix of carbs, fats and proteins in a natural manner.

Use the table below to select the various components of your thali. The table has a list of commonly eaten food items for lunch and dinner, but is by no means an exhaustive list, so feel free to add in more items of your preference. I have divided the list into proteins, grains, and vegetables. As per the 1:2:3 plan, select items to put into your thali. Each portion size is close to 100 calories, making it a 600-calorie meal. The serving size is one medium vati, the kind we usually use in our homes. Also, besides each item, the amount of proteins per serving is also mentioned. Be conscious of the number, and make sure you try and get between 15 to 20 grams per meal.

Make your own thali. Select 1:2:3 from the groups below

Proteins (select one)	Portion	Protein (g)
Vegetarian options		
Soya nuggets	1 vati	10.0
Kadhi	1 vati*	3.2
Punjabi dal (or mixed dal)	1 vati	7.0
Peas	1 vati	5.8
Chhole	1 vati	6.0
Green moong sprouts	1 vati	7.0
Paneer bhurji	1 vati**	9.5
Paneer tikka	2-3 medium-sized cubes	7.0
Curd (made with cow's milk)	1 vati*	3.2
Non-vegetarian options		
1 whole egg + 1 white	1 egg and 1 egg white	9.5
Egg whites	3 eggs	9.0
Grilled fish (palm size)	1 piece	20.0
Chicken tikka (boneless)	4-5 medium pieces	26.0
Chicken breast	1	20.0

Grains (select two)	Portion	Protein (g)
Whole-wheat roti	2 medium	3.6
Multigrain bread	2 slices**	3.6
Bajra bhakri	1 medium, thick	3.5
Idli	2 medium/ 3 small	3.5
Pasta (without white sauce)	1 medium vati (8-10 pcs)	3.4
White bread	2 slcs	3.1
Upma/poha	1 vati	2.5
Brown rice	1 vati	1.8

Kurmura	1 vati*	1.1
White rice (cooked)	1 heaped vati	1.9
VEGETABLES (SELECT THREE)	PORTION	PROTEIN (G)
Palak paneer	1 vati*	2.5
Soya nuggets and capsicum	1 vati	3.2
Stir-fry (corn, mushroom, capsicum/broccoli/tofu)	1 vati*	2.0
Beetroot raita	1 vati	2.5
Peas and cauliflower subzi	1 vati	3.0
Cabbage subzi	1 vati*	1.0
Pav bhaji (w/o butter)	1 vati	1.0
Mix leafy vegetables	1 vati	1.5
Potato subzi	1 vati	1.0
Raw banana subzi	1 vati	1.0

*Less than 80 cal; **More than 120 cal

Principle No. 2

Focus on vegetables and fruits

The benefits of vegetables and fruits have been unequivocally established. They tend to be high in nutrients and low in calories. They are also great sources of vitamins, minerals, antioxidants and dietary fibre. The majority of Indians are vegetarians, and this advice sounds easy to follow, but there is a big difference between being vegetarian and eating fruits and vegetables. In fact, various surveys have shown that the amount of fruit and vegetable consumption in our diet tends to be very low.

Cereals and pulses form the majority of the Indian diet. Even when vegetables are included, they are often overcooked in a large quantity of oil or ghee. In the process of overheating and deep frying, most of the nutrient content is lost, and though you are eating the vegetable, you are not deriving the benefit. On the other hand, you are greatly increasing your oil intake, and if this oil is re-used, then it is even more detrimental to your health.

In terms of which fruits and vegetables to select, remember the ones that are richly coloured are better, since they tend to be higher in vitamins and minerals. Good examples are spinach, carrots, tomatoes and peas. Tomatoes are rich in lycopene, an antioxidant which is beneficial in reducing prostate cancer in men. Did you know that technically tomato is considered a fruit and not a vegetable? Don't worry, I didn't know either, until my 11-year-old daughter pointed it out to me! Beetroot is another great choice, since it is rich in nitrates. Nitrates release a substance called nitric oxide in the arteries. Nitric oxide helps to relax the arteries, lower blood pressure and improve blood flow to the heart.

Your recommended quantity of vegetables and fruits will depend on your total caloric need, but in general it is recommended to eat five to eight servings of fruits and vegetables per day. These can be obtained from three portions eaten at lunch, three at dinner, and two fruits eaten as snacks during the day.

Fruits

Many people are averse to eating fruit but will happily gulp down juices, thinking them to be the elixir of life. In Mumbai, several eateries have made their name on the popularity of their fruit juices, which usually cost more than the food served there. My opinion on fruit juices is a bit mixed. A lot depends on the manner in which the juice is made, and for that I would mainly look at the amount of sugar added to the juice. If there isn't any, then that's a plus. However, even if there isn't any added sugar, there are two reasons why it's always better to eat the fruit rather than drink the juice. The first has to do with calories. Let's consider the case of the most popular fruit juice in our country, mosambi (sweet lime) juice. To make a glass, you need to squeeze at least three sweet limes, if not four. On the other hand, if you eat the fruit, it's unlikely that you will eat more than one, or at the most two, before you feel satisfied. By drinking the juice, you effectively consume double the calories. The second reason is fibre. Most fruits contain plenty of fibre, but when we make juice out of them, the fibre is often lost. Soluble fibre present in fruit is extremely beneficial in keeping your blood cholesterol under control. Therefore, it's always better to eat the fruit rather than drink the juice. This does not mean that you should never have juice, but it's important to be aware of what you are consuming. Once there is awareness, you will be able to regulate your intake to match your body's requirements. On the subject of juices, I would recommend that you restrict consumption of packaged juices to a minimum. Besides some of the drawbacks we discussed, packaged juices tend to contain a lot of added sugar as well.

What about non-vegetarian food?

This is another area of controversy in the world of nutrition (are there any non-controversial areas, you may well ask). Opinions range from telling heart patients to follow a completely vegetarian diet on the one hand, and on the other, diets such as the 'Paleo' diet are gaining popularity. Paleo is a short form of Palaeolithic, and as the name suggests, the diet is based on what our forefathers ate when they were still cavemen. It is also popularly referred to as the stone-age or hunter-gatherer diet, and encourages the consumption of meat. In my opinion, chicken and fish can be included as part of a heart-healthy diet, but should not form the major portion of your plate. Red meat and processed meat on the other hand are associated with a higher risk for heart disease, and certain types of cancer, especially colorectal cancer. Red meat includes beef, mutton, and lamb. That does not mean that you can never eat them, but they should not be eaten frequently. If you were to eat them a few times a month, in a limited quantity (size of a deck of cards), that would be fine.

Principle No. 3

Make it complex

Carbohydrates are the main source of energy and can broadly be divided into simple and complex. Simple carbohydrates, also known as sugars, help in providing instant energy. Over the years, when dieters have tried to cut the fat in their diet, they have replaced it with sugars, which also contain calories. When taken in excess they get converted to triglycerides in the blood, which increases your total cholesterol level and risk for heart disease. The largest source of simple sugars for most people tends to come from soft drinks, juices, and the addition of sugar to coffee or tea. In addition, sweets such as cakes, cookies, ice creams and mithai have a high amount of sugars added to them. In nutrition terms we call these 'empty calories', since they increase weight and have no health benefits. I do not recommend that you stop eating or drinking these items completely, but you should be aware that they are high sources of sugar, and should be taken in moderation.

Fruits also contain simple sugars, but in addition have vitamins, minerals, and fibre and should not be avoided. A lot of other foods which we consume regularly, such as milk products and refined flour, also contain a fair amount of sugar. Some of them have sugar naturally present, while some have sugar added to them. It's the added sugars which tend to be a problem. There are a wide variety of sugars which are added to commercial food products, and you should look for them on food labels. Some of the more common ones are sucrose, fructose, maltose and corn syrup. You should avoid food products that have these listed as their first ingredient, which suggests that they are the primary ingredient in the food. In the Indian context, we tend not to have a lot of processed items, but the largest culprit is probably the sugar we add in our beverages, along with the sweets made at home. Many people believe that substituting honey or jaggery for sugar is a better option. Both of them do have some health attributes, which sugar doesn't, but at the end of the day they are very similar in composition to sugar and I would advise you to keep their use to a minimum.

Complex carbohydrates are made up of three or more simple sugars linked together. They are commonly referred to as starches. They take longer to digest, since they first need to be broken to simple sugars before the body absorbs them. Common dietary sources include roti, brown rice, starchy vegetables such as potatoes, spinach, beans and whole-wheat bread. A practical method of including complex carbs in your diet is to use different whole grains for rotis, and to replace white rice and bread for brown rice and whole-wheat bread. The term brown bread can sometimes be misleading, since some bakeries just colour it brown and it's not genuinely a whole grain product. This reminds me of a popular diet in which you are told to avoid everything white, such as salt, sugar, white rice and white bread. It's considered poison for your body. I would not go so far as to call it poison, but it is a good idea to have more brown products than white.

A few years ago, I had gone to a rural area to conduct a health camp, and after a long morning of seeing patients, my team and I were taking a well-deserved lunch break. The food was laid out on separate tables for doctors and local area volunteers. On the doctors' table were hot, fluffy naans, which a volunteer proudly informed me were sourced from a restaurant in a town some distance away. On the volunteers' table were coarse-looking rotis which were made at home, using bajra. The locals were aghast when I asked if I could eat the bajra rotis instead of the naans. Naans are made of refined flour, and are far inferior to unrefined grains such as bajra, ragi or jowar, which contain a large amount of complex carbs. It's one of the tragedies of life that as we get richer our diet gets poorer.

Fibre

Dietary fibre is commonly known as roughage. It is a type of carbohydrate which cannot be digested by the body. It passes through the digestive system and is removed from the body without adding any calories. Soluble fibre dissolves in water and is found commonly in fruits and oats. It helps to lower blood glucose and cholesterol. Insoluble fibre is found in whole-wheat flour, wheat bran, beans and vegetables. It helps provide bulk to the stools, and thereby in relieving constipation. Adding it to your diet will help you start your day with a 'clean' stomach. Research has shown that a diet high in fibre lowers your risk for heart disease, colon cancer and several other gastrointestinal diseases. You should aim to get between 25–35 grams of fibre in your daily diet.

Fibre content of food per serving size

Food item	Portion size	Soluble fibre (g)	Insoluble fibre (g)	Total fibre (g)
Chickoo	1 medium size	1.4	6.8	**8.2**
Rajma sabzi	1 vati	3.0	3.0	**6.0**
Bran wheat flakes	1 vati	0.5	4.5	**5.0**
Pear	1 medium size	3.0	2.0	**5.0**
Sprouted moong (soaked)	1 vati	0.6	4.1	**4.7**
Dry dates	4-5 pcs	0.7	3.5	**4.2**
Apple	1 medium size	1.0	3.0	**4.0**
Muesli (with nuts)	1 vati, 3 tbsp	0.6	3.1	**3.7**
Dalia (broken wheat), cooked	1 vati	0.9	2.8	**3.7**
French beans subzi	1 vati	2.4	1.3	**3.7**
Oatmeal (cooked)	1 vati	1.3	2.2	**3.5**
Carrots, raw	1 medium size	1.0	2.5	**3.5**
Methi leaves subzi	1 vati	1.1	2.4	**3.5**
Dal	1 vati	0.6	2.5	**3.1**
Palak subzi	1 vati	1.0	2.0	**3.0**
Broccoli (partially cooked)	1 vati	1.5	1.5	**3.0**
Banana	1 medium sized	1.0	2.0	**3.0**
Bajra roti	1 large bhakri	0.5	1.8	**2.3**
Brown rice (cooked)	1 vati	Trace	2.0	**2.0**
Almonds	10-12 pcs	0.6	1.3	**1.9**

Principle No. 4

Watch the fat

The pendulum on fat seems to keep swinging every few years. There are diets which consider fats to be taboo, and there are other diets which advocate eating fat in large amounts. In reality, as is usually the case, the truth lies somewhere between. Fats do form part of a healthy diet, but need to be consumed in moderation, which could be anywhere from 20–30 per cent of your daily intake. More important than total fat intake is the nature of fat consumed, with saturated fat clearly being the villain. Your total intake of saturated fat should definitely be below 10 per cent of your dietary intake.

In the '90s, dietary fat was thought to be public enemy number one (just as eggs were in the '80s) and manufacturers went overboard to reduce the quantity of fat in their packaged foods. They cut out the fat in their products, but to compensate for the drop in taste, they substituted it with sugar and salt. These sugars were almost inevitably simple sugars, which consequently led to an increase in triglycerides as well as weight. When I was living in the US, I remember walking home from university and seeing my roommate Shane with a large bag of chips in his hand. He clearly intended to finish the packet and on seeing my look of disbelief, he proudly informed me that they were 'fat-free'. Shane and several millions like him soon discovered that fat-free did not translate to calorie-free, and though the US went through a period in which dietary fat consumption was reduced, their weight and waistline continued expanding. They simply made up the fat calories through sugars. What's more, the 'fat-free' label lulled consumers into a sense of false confidence, and led them to consume more of the product than they would its full fat version.

Dieticians often refer to visible and invisible fats. Visible fats are literally those which are visible, such as oil, ghee, and butter. Invisible fats are present in food products which we often don't think of as containing fat. For example, cereals are thought of as pure carbs, but they do contain some amount of fat. Similarly, pulses too contain some amount of fat. Since we get a fair amount of fat in our diet without realizing it, I advocate using oil, ghee and butter in limited amounts. Total consumption of these should be between 1–1.5 tablespoons per person per day. You can read more about it in the section on oils.

Saturated fat content in food, per serving size

Food item	Serving size	Saturated fat (g)
Full fat buffalo milk	1 glass (240 ml)	7.5
Butter cookies	2 pieces	6.6
Processed cheese	1 cube	6.3
Butter	1 tbsp	6.1
Lamb meat	3-5 pieces	6
Ice cream	1 large scoop	6
Fried potato vada	1 vada	5.4*
Milk prepared from whole milk powder	2 tbsp; 1 glass milk	5.1
Milk chocolate	2 small squares	4.8
Oatmeal cookies	2 pieces	4.8
Full fat cow's milk	1 glass	3.5
Whole egg	1	2.8
Gulab jamun	2 med pieces	2.4*
Chicken, without skin	1 leg piece	2.2
Double-toned milk	1 glass	2
Paneer	2-3 med cubes	1.7
Potato chips	1 packet	1.4*
Cashew nuts	7-8	1.2
Tea-biscuits	2 biscuits	1.2

*can contain trans-fats

Cholesterol

If you were to walk into an American supermarket in the '90s and you were given a dollar each time you read the phrase 'cholesterol-free', you would have gotten rich very quickly. Today, however, you don't read that phrase quite that often, not because cholesterol is any less important, but because we have a better understanding of cholesterol production in our body. Until 50 years ago, we really were not too clued-in on the importance of cholesterol as a risk factor for heart disease. Since then, nutritionists and food manufacturers have been on a witch hunt for cholesterol in food products, and have tried all means to get rid of it. The interesting thing is that cholesterol is only found in food of animal origin. Hypothetically, therefore, vegetarians should not get any cholesterol in their diet, except through milk, which is an 'animal product'. Then why do vegetarians suffer from high cholesterol too?

Think of your liver as a factory in which cholesterol production takes place. The saturated fat that we consume in our diet is converted to cholesterol in the liver. Many vegetarian diets tend to be high in saturated fat, which explains why vegetarians do not have immunity to high cholesterol levels. Interestingly, the cholesterol in the food that we eat is not converted to the cholesterol in our blood to the same degree as saturated fat is.

Foods which are rich in cholesterol, like the yellow of an egg and shell fish (such as shrimp or prawns), are considered taboo foods by most cardiologists and nutritionists. However, both of these are actually quite low in saturated fat and therefore when eaten in moderate quantities can be part of a heart-healthy diet. Like in all things, a sense of balance needs to prevail. So, on a day when you have had an egg or two for breakfast, it would be wise to curtail your shrimp intake and vice-versa. Organ meats such as liver, kidney, and brain are unusually high in cholesterol, and should be consumed very sparingly, if at all.

Which oil should you use?

Remember that all oils are made up of fat, but they have them in different components as discussed earlier—monounsaturated or MUFA, polyunsaturated or PUFA, and saturated fat. Saturated fats are converted to cholesterol in the body, and therefore oils high in this should be avoided. Typically, coconut oil, palm oil and ghee have the highest amount of saturated fat. Now, you may have heard several naturopathy practitioners advocate the virtues of coconut oil and ghee, but to be honest I am not aware of any large-scale studies done with the necessary scientific rigour, which have borne out these claims. That is not to suggest that they may not work, it's just that the evidence is not out there at the moment. If they are consumed in a small quantity as part of an overall heart-healthy diet, then they should not cause any harm. By small quantity, I mean a teaspoon a day of either.

Most advertisements for oils usually have the words 'cholesterol-free' emblazoned across them. While this is technically true, I personally feel it's a bit misleading. As explained a little earlier, cholesterol is only present in animal products. Oils are a vegetable product, and by default are cholesterol-free. Therefore, putting a big label proclaiming it is to imply that particular oil is the only one which is free of cholesterol, when in reality all oils are cholesterol-free.

One of the questions I am asked most often is which oil should be used, and there is no single correct answer to that one. Most studies have looked at olive oil and found it an excellent option, but at the same time one has to bear in mind that those same studies usually looked at the Mediterranean diet as opposed to olive oil in isolation. A lot of the health benefits were due to the overall diet composition, and not just the virtue of the oil.

Olive oil is very high in MUFA, as is canola oil, which is a modified rapeseed oil. This seed is primarily grown in Canada, and hence the name. Canola is high in MUFA and very low in saturated fats and is a good choice. One advantage of canola oil over olive oil is that it withstands high heat better, which would suit our Indian style of cooking. Canola oil is also one of the few oils that is rich in omega-3 fatty acids, which are beneficial for the heart.

Among the commonly used oils in India, groundnut oil is high in MUFA, as is mustard oil.

A recent trend is to manufacture blended oils. Rice bran oil is popular in several Asian countries, and is being used increasingly in India. It has been blended with other PUFA-rich oils and studies have shown it to be beneficial in reducing cholesterol as part of an overall heart-healthy diet.

I believe that most oils are fine to use, as long as the quantity is controlled. I recommend three teaspoons (which equals one tablespoon or 15 ml) of oil per person per day. This roughly translates to half a kilo or litre of oil per person per month. This also assumes that all your meals are home-cooked.

If only half your meals are from home, then you need to reduce the quantity in half.

Of late, dieticians have been advocating a mix and match approach, in which you rotate cooking oils and use a different one each time the current bottle is over. That might not be a bad idea, but you would need to maintain a large inventory at home. Another approach is to match the oil to the type of cooking. For example, an olive oil perfectly complements a salad, while groundnut or canola oil can be used to cook vegetables at a high flame.

Fatty acid composition of vegetable oils and fats (expressed as a percentage of total fatty acid content: MUFA – monounsaturated fatty acid; PUFA – polyunsaturated fatty acid)

Type of oil	Sat fat (per cent)	MUFA (per cent)	PUFA (per cent)	
			OMEGA 3	OMEGA 6
Canola oil	7	61	11	21
Flaxseed oil	9	18	57	16
Sunflower oil	12	16	1	71
Corn oil	13	29	1	57
Olive oil	14	73	Trace	13
Soybean oil	15	23	8	54
Groundnut oil	19	48	Trace	33
Rice bran oil	22.1	41	1.4	34.3
Cottonseed oil	27	19	Trace	54
Vanaspati	46	49.4	-	4.4
Palm oil	51	39	Trace	10
Ghee	65	32	-	3
Butter	68	28	1	3
Coconut oil	91	7	-	2

Trans-fat

The world of fats is full of acronyms, such as MUFA and PUFA, and if that were not confusing enough, there is another type of fat called trans-fat.

Trans-fat is made by adding hydrogen to vegetable oil through a process called hydrogenation. It is a type of unsaturated fat which makes the oil less likely to spoil. It is widely used in the food manufacturing industry, since it helps increase the shelf-life of food products. While it does increase the shelf-life of food products, it has been shown to decrease human life and is considered the most dangerous type of fat by most doctors. Trans-fat increases LDL cholesterol and decreases HDL cholesterol, which is a double whammy. When you read a food label, look out for the ingredient 'partially hydrogenated vegetable oil', another term for trans-fat.

The recommendation is to consume as little trans-fat as possible in your food, and consequently there is no recommended daily limit. Scandinavian countries, which are famous for having the best health indicators for their population, have taken the lead and banned the use of trans-fat in commercial foods. Several world cities and countries have also banned or reduced the quantity of trans-fat in prepared foods. Closer home, many biscuit manufacturers have chosen to voluntarily cut out trans-fats from their biscuits (usually a high source of trans-fats in the Indian diet).

Principle No. 5

Size matters—calorie and weight control

Research on different types of diets has thrown up conflicting results, but one thing is clear: size does matter, your body size that is. Across all research it has been clearly demonstrated that a healthy weight is key for good health. While that sounds overly simplistic, it's important to make a few clarifications at this point. A healthy weight is key to good health, but that does not mean that you automatically enjoy good health based just on your weight. Your overall lifestyle, which includes diet and exercise, needs to be good as well. On the other hand, there are a large number of people who are overweight and have adopted healthy lifestyles and shown great improvements in their metabolic parameters (such as sugar and cholesterol), even if they continue to remain overweight, the so-called 'fat and fit' category.

The first step in planning a healthy diet is to figure out which weight category you fall in. Obesity is defined as excess body fat. There are several different ways to measure body fat, and each has its pros and cons. Currently, the most universally accepted method is the body mass index (BMI) method, which is calculated by dividing your weight in kilograms, by your height (expressed in metre square). Based on this, you need to figure out which BMI category you fall into. (Refer to BMI chart in the chapter, Risk Factors). If you are overweight or obese, you need to set medium and long-term goals for weight loss. It is important that these goals are realistic, and are discussed in detail in the chapter on weight loss.

I was recently at a seminar on marathon running in Goa, and one of my co-panellists was Ryan Fernando. Ryan is a nutritionist and biochemist with an entrepreneurial streak, and runs a chain of successful nutrition clinics in Bangalore and Chennai. When I first met him, two things immediately stood out. First, he was a male nutritionist, and second was the fact that he had a BMI well below 21 kg/m^2, which one doesn't see too often in nutritionists!

Ryan started his talk by saying that he always advised clients to eat to their heart's content. Just as the audience heaved a sigh of relief, he put his fist up in the air, and reminded us all that our heart is the size of our fist. So, we needed to eat only that much. I thought that was a beautiful analogy, and brought home the message that portion and calorie control are very important. People are often under the mistaken assumption that as long as they eat the 'right' food, quantity does not matter.

How much do you currently eat?

The best way to calculate how much you eat is to maintain a detailed food diary for three days. You need to record everything that you eat from the moment you wake up till you are back in bed at night. For greater accuracy, carry a small diary, or should I say smart phone, and record in it as soon as you eat. Don't wait till night to try and recollect your entire day's food intake, or you may forget that peda your office colleague gave you at noon to celebrate the birth of his kid, or the chocolate your son shared with you just before dinner. Write it down as soon as you finish eating it. Make sure you include one weekend day in the three days, since your eating pattern is usually different on weekends. After you finish, show it to a dietician who can then analyze it for you, and make a report on your calorie, carb, fat, and protein consumption.

Suresh Mehta was 80 years old when he won the prestigious Mercedes Golf Cup at the Willingdon Club in Mumbai, in 2010. This was in addition to several other tournaments he had won in his career, in Mumbai and Coimbatore. Mr Mehta had always led a healthy lifestyle, and so the need for bypass surgery in 2004 came to him as a rude shock. He belonged to the 5 per cent who did everything correct but still suffered, though it was

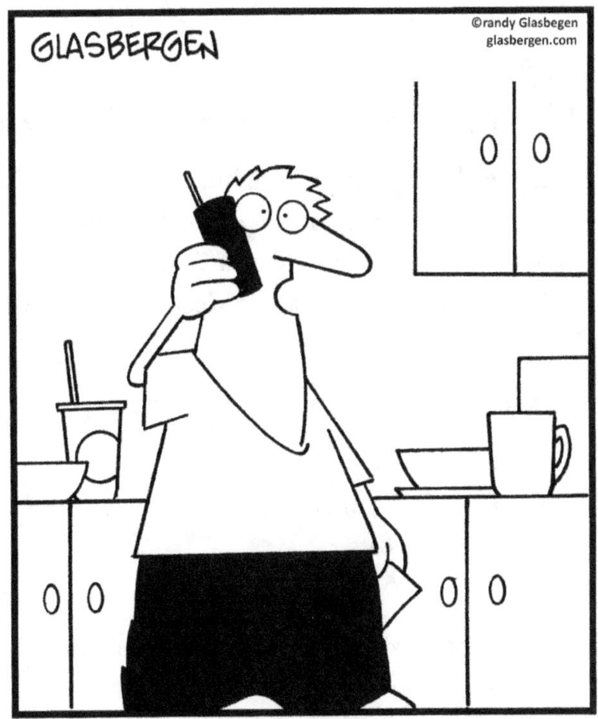

**"Don't slice the pizza. My diet says
I'm only allowed to eat one piece!"**

at the age of 74. After surgery, he was determined to get back to his active lifestyle and told me that he was ready to do what it took for him to speed up his recovery.

When talking about nutrition, I stressed the importance of portion control and total calories. I asked him to fill in a three-day food chart to analyze how much he ate. I was pleasantly surprised when he came back with a neatly typed A-4 sheet which had all the details of what he had eaten. To the nearest gram! He had actually weighed every bit of food that he consumed, and had also brought along a roti to show me the average diameter and thickness of the roti he ate. In all my years of seeing patients, this was the first time I'd seen this level of precision. Maybe that's why he achieved one more spectacular feat of precision in golf—he has got seven hole-in-ones during his career, which as any golfer will tell you is extremely rare.

How much should you eat?

Follow these three simple steps to calculate your daily calorie requirement.

1. Calculate your weight in pounds. Weight in pounds = weight in kg x 2.2
2. Calculate your metabolic rate (BMR) = weight in pounds x 10
3. If you are sedentary multiply BMR by 1.2; if you are active (exercising for at least 30 minutes, three days a week) then multiply BMR by 1.5.

The final answer is your daily caloric requirement.

Example: for a 70 kg sedentary person
Weight in pounds = 154 pounds
BMR = 154 x 10 = 1540 cals
For a sedentary person: 1540 x 1.2 = 1848 cals.

This is the daily caloric requirement for weight maintenance. Naturally, if you want to lose weight, you will need to eat less than this amount.

How often should you eat?

While growing up, I was always taught to be disciplined about my eating. The prevalent thought was that one should eat at mealtimes, and nothing between. Now, the thinking is almost the opposite. Dieticians recommend eating frequent small meals, with many suggesting six meals a day, and some suggesting that you eat every two hours. I am not sure how practical it is to eat every two hours, especially if you are working, and are not the boss of the company. I would recommend splitting your daily food consumption into three main meals of the day, accompanied by two snacks. Breakfast, lunch and dinner are your main meals, and in addition you should have a mid-morning and mid-evening snack. About 60 per cent of your calories could be divided between lunch and dinner, and 40 per cent between breakfast and snacks. This combination is both healthy and practical. Here is a sample break-up of the day for a person consuming a 2,000 calorie diet:

- Breakfast: 8 a.m. – 300 calories
- Mid-morning snack: 10:30 a.m. – 250 calories
- Lunch: 1 p.m. – 600 calories
- Mid-evening snack: 4-5 p.m. – 250 calories
- Dinner: 8 p.m. – 600 calories

The table below lists some healthy breakfast and snack options. You can mix and match such that it totals 250–300 calories. Also, pay attention to protein, and try and get in 5–10 grams of protein in your breakfast, mid-morning and mid-evening snack.

Breakfast and snack options

Options	Serving size	Calories (cal)	Protein (g)
Oatmeal porridge with nuts (glass of milk+ 3 tbsp of oats + 2 walnuts, 4 almonds + 1-2 dates)	1 bowl	250	9.7
Egg omelette with vegetables (1 whole egg + 1 white+ ½ tsp oil + tomatoes, onion, mushrooms, spinach)	1 omelette	127	9.5
Poha with vegetables (carrot, French beans, beetroot)	1 large vati	150	2.8
2 dry bajra khakras with sprouts	2 medium sized + 1 vati	265	8.1
Green moong chilla (½ tsp oil)	1 medium	98	5.3
Sandwich (2 slices multigrain bread + 1 tbsp hummus + vegetables— lettuce, tomatoes, cucumber, beetroot)	1 sandwich	200	6.0
Dry bhel with vegetables and sprouts (without sev or puri)	1 large vati	150	3.2
Steamed vegetable idlis (carrot, beans, beetroot) with sambhar	2 medium sized + 1 vati	240	5.8
Paneer and vegetable roll (homemade low-fat paneer + tomatoes, red cabbage, spring onions, lettuce and hung curd dressing)	1 roll	220	10.0
Almonds (8-10) and 2 whole walnuts	10 + 2	100	3.5
Fruit (1 medium apple, pear, orange, 3 slices papaya)	1 large vati mixed fruit	65-75	1.0
Multigrain bread	2 slices	140	3.0
A glass of milk or thick butter milk	1 glass	100	4.8
Tea/coffee with 1 tsp sugar and toned milk	1 cup	53	1.6

Other dietary aspects

The five principles that we've discussed above should be the foundation of your diet. If you are able to follow these closely, you will certainly be on the path of prevention and reversal of heart disease. However, I am sure you still have a hundred questions on areas which we have not yet touched. Can I eat salt? How much? What about milk, is it good for you or bad for you? Can I eat spices? In the rest of the chapter, I will touch upon those areas of nutrition that I'm most often questioned about by patients. Of course, it probably won't answer every food-related question you have, but should certainly be enough food for thought. And then you have Google!

Diet for diabetics

My father-in-law's brother has been diabetic since childhood. Every time we go to their house for a meal, I have seen meat and vegetables piled up in his plate. If anyone even by mistake offers a piece of bread or roti to him, his sister gets upset and reminds them that he is diabetic. I think the single biggest misconception in nutrition is that diabetics cannot eat rice, bread or rotis. Actually, if you read the dietary recommendations of the major diabetic associations all over the world, you will notice that they are pretty much the same as those recommended for 'normal' people. Carbohydrates are not poison food, and should be consumed as part of a diabetic-friendly diet. The fear has been that carbs are made up of sugar and they will cause the blood sugar levels to increase. All carbs are not the same, and they vary in their ability to raise blood sugar. The glycemic index (GI) measures how much a particular food causes blood sugar to rise. Therefore foods with high GI will raise your blood sugar level rapidly, and should be eaten less frequently for those with diabetes. A GI of less than 55 is considered low, 55–70 is medium while more than 70 is considered high. White rice, white bread, potato, and sugar are foods with a high GI. On the other hand, beans, lentils, milk and whole grains typically have a low GI.

In the recent past, sugar has received so much attention that entire diets are planned around the GI status of foods. However, the GI does not give the full picture, since the actual 'sugar-raising capability' of the food will also depend on the amount consumed. The glycemic load (GL) takes into account the GI of the food as well as the typical quantity of the food, and in many ways is more important. You will be happy to know that ice-cream has a high GI, but a low GL, so can certainly be part of a healthy diet when eaten occasionally (assuming you eat only one scoop, of course).

GL = GI (of the food) x amount of the food eaten in gms / 100

It's important to remember that the total carbohydrate content eaten during the day has far more bearing on the blood sugar of a diabetic as opposed to individual food items. Check the table below for the GI as well as GL of commonly-eaten foods. Remember, a food low in GI will still raise your sugars if eaten in larger than normal quantities, and a food high in GI is acceptable if consumed in restricted amounts. A glycemic load of 10 or below is considered good, while above 20 is considered high.

Glycemic index and glycemic load of commonly-eaten foods

FOOD PRODUCT	GI	SERVING SIZE	GL
White rice (cooked)	89	1 vati	34
Instant oatmeal with milk	83	1 large vati	22
Potato subzi	76	1 large	26
Watermelon	72	5-6 cubes	4
Pineapple	68	4 slcs	6
Basmati, white rice (cooked)	67	1 heaped vati	22
Upma	67	1 vati	22
Muesli (w/o raisins)	66	2 heaped tbsp	13
Cornflakes with 125ml milk	65	2 heaped tbsp	19
Cream cracker biscuits (no sugar)	65	2 biscuits	11
Banana	62	1 large	16
Honey	61	1 tbsp	7
Idli	60	3 medium pcs	19
Muesli fruit & nut	59	2 heaped tbsp	19

Food product	GI	Serving size	GL
Ice-cream	57	1 medium scoop	7
Papaya	56	1 large vati	5
Dosa	55	1 large	22
Bran wheat flakes	55	2 heaped tbsp	14
Boiled peas	51	1 vati	4
Brown rice (cooked)	50	1 heaped vati	13
Chapatti, multigrain atta	49	2 medium roti	15
Bajra roti	49	2 small	10
Milk chocolate	49	2 small squares	7
Moong cheela	45	2 medium pcs	22
Dates	42	5 pcs	18
Orange	33	1 medium sized	3
Carrot subzi	33	1 vati	2
Yellow dal (thick)	29	1 vati	3
Apple	29	1 medium sized	6
Pear	28	1 medium sized	5
Dark chocolate	23	1 large square	3
Mixed dry fruits	21	¾ vati	3
Cow's milk	21	1 large glass	3
Rajma subzi	19	1 vati	11
Buffalo milk	11	1 large glass	1
Chole subzi (kabuli chana)	10	1 vati	6

- Low GI < 55
- Moderate GI 55-70
- High GI > 70
- Low GL < 10
- High GL ≥ 10

Artificial sweeteners (sugar substitutes)

Artificial sweeteners, often referred to as sugar substitutes, are compounds that add sweetness without calories. Their level of sweetness is several times that of sugar, so a very small amount is needed. The most common artificial sweeteners used are saccharin (Sweet 'n Low), aspartame (Equal or NutraSweet), and sucralose (Splenda). Today, they are used in a host of products, including chocolates, soft drinks, chewing gums, yogurt and ice-cream. They have two advantages. They provide sweetness to food without raising blood sugar. This is a great boon for diabetics who have been using them for decades, especially as sugar substitutes in their tea or coffee. The other advantage is that they are calorie-free.

While they are extremely popular, they have not been without their fair share of controversy. In the 1970s, a study linked bladder cancer in rats with saccharin, sparking off a scare, which has to some extent remained till present. However, further studies have shown that this risk did not translate to humans, and several subsequent studies have not linked artificial sweeteners with any serious health concerns. Of late, another concern has been raised that artificial sweeteners actually lead to weight gain, rather than weight loss. It is theorised that these sweeteners do not satisfy the sweet cravings in the brain, and people taking them end up eating more than usual.

Here is my take on artificial sweeteners. If you are diabetic and are comfortable eliminating added sugar from your diet, then that's the best option. However, if you do like using sweeteners, go ahead and use them, but moderately, which means up to a few packets a day added to your coffee or tea. The safe upper limit of their use is very high, and it's difficult to cross it with normal consumption. If you are using them as a way to cut calories, keep their use to a minimum, since the dust has not yet settled on the weight gain controversy.

Also, bear in mind that because a product is 'sugar-free', it does not mean it's calorie free. Just as it happened for fats in the 1990s, the trend today is to have sugar-free products, but many of them (with the exception of most diet drinks) do have calories from other sources. The danger is that you may eat it in excess, and at the end of the day, consume more calories than you would have if normal sugar was present.

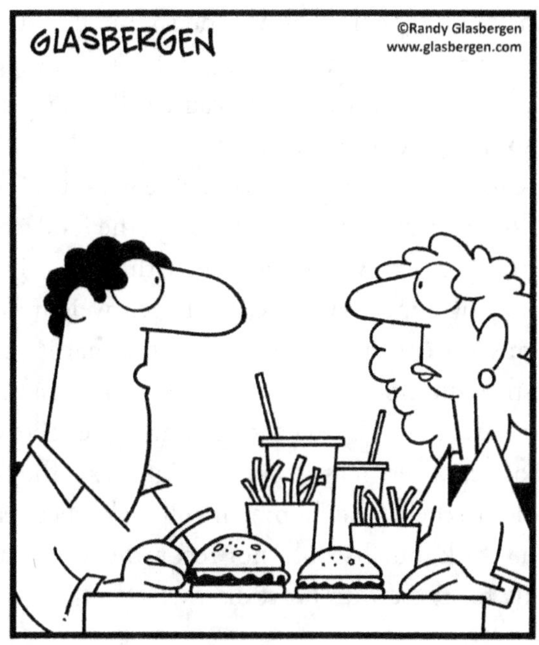

"Fast food is a dieter's worst enemy...
but my mother taught me to love my enemies!"

Water

Water is vital for the optimal functioning of the body, and is considered a macronutrient (nutrient required in large quantity), but what is not quite certain is the exact amount required per person. Water forms about 60 per cent of our body weight, and helps transport nutrients to various parts of the body, as well as flush out toxins. We have been taught since childhood to consume at least eight glasses of water per day, which roughly equals two litres of water. Your need for water depends on factors, such as environmental conditions. In the hot and humid conditions that we often experience in India, your need for water increases. At the same time, a lot of people believe in the detoxifying properties of water and consciously drink upwards of four litres per day. I am unsure of any benefit of water consumption in excess of your body requirements. The colour of your urine is a good guide to your hydration status. Ideally it should be colourless or a light yellow colour.

Dark yellow urine indicates dehydration, and should be corrected as soon as possible. At this point, it's important to remember that certain medications, especially some of the B vitamins, tend to cause yellow discolouration of the urine, due to colouring agents in the capsule.

Besides drinking water, the food we consume is a source of water, and up to 20 per cent of our water intake comes through the food we eat. Fruits and vegetables tend to have high water content, with some—like watermelons and tomatoes—having almost 90 per cent of their weight as water.

One of the misconceptions regarding water is that it contains calories. Water is calorie-free and no matter how much you consume, you will not put on weight because of it. Having a lot of water does give you a feeling of fullness, so a lot of people use it as an aid to weight loss. They consume water a few minutes prior to their meal, hoping it will make them eat less. To some extent this might work, but I would not recommend this as a weight-loss strategy, especially for those with heart disease.

Water and heart disease

This may come as a surprise to many, but for some heart patients, excess water can actually be detrimental. Patients with a low ejection fraction (heart-pumping capacity) suffer from heart failure, a condition in which the heart is not able to pump adequate blood to meet the demands of the body. As mentioned earlier, a normal ejection fraction (EF) is 55-65 per cent, and it's considered low when it drops below 35 per cent. When there is fluid overload in the body, the heart has to work harder to pump blood at the required pressure. In a normal heart it does not matter, but in a weak heart this will lead to further strain and possible damage. In fact, for both blood pressure and heart failure cases, we often prescribe a class of drugs called diuretics, also known as water pills. The purpose of these drugs is to remove excess fluid from the body. Therefore, rather than take in excess fluid and then load up on medications to get rid of it, it makes sense to control intake in the first place. If you have a low EF, it is suggested to restrict your fluid intake to 1.5 litres a day, which includes liquids like tea, coffee, milk, cold drinks and soups. This amount may be increased or decreased depending upon your individual condition. It's also a good idea to weigh yourself daily if you have heart failure. An increase in more than 1 kg over a 24-hour period, or 3 kg in a week, is a sign that you may be retaining fluid and you should talk to your doctor. Excess fluid in the body, especially the lungs, tends to cause breathlessness, and is not a good sign.

Water during exercise

It is important to increase your water consumption when exercising, especially outdoors. Earlier the recommendation was to consume as much as possible during exercise, but new research has shown that there is something such as too much water. Excess water tends to dilute the sodium content in the body, leading to a dangerous condition called hyponatremia (low sodium). The best advice is to adjust your water intake depending on your sweat rate. We are in the midst of conducting a sweat-rate study on the Indian population to determine the average sweat loss during an hour of outdoor exercise. The initial results have thrown up interesting readings, with sweat rates varying from half a litre to almost three litres per hour.

I was the Medical Director of the Standard Chartered Mumbai Marathon, and during the 2011 race, I got a call that a runner had collapsed. I dashed off to the spot, and when I saw the runner, I was shocked since it was my good friend Pulin Shroff. We quickly transported him to our base camp and rehydrated him with intravenous solutions. Almost two years later, when Pulin took part in the sweat study, his sweat rate was at the high end of the spectrum, upwards of two litres per hour. That helped explain what happened on that Sunday in 2011, and I am sure Pulin will now pay special attention to his hydration while exercising.

What about milk?

I think two consumer items that Indians hold very dear to their heart are milk and gold. There is no connection between the two, except for the fact that there is huge adulteration in both. For the moment, I will assume that you have a heart of gold (unadulterated), and focus only on milk.

Milk is a topic that evokes huge scientific and emotional debate, since there are several aspects to its consumption, ranging from health concerns to ethics. From a health perspective there is a fierce debate on the benefits and ills of milk and dairy products, with opinions swinging wildly on both ends. In the Indian context, milk is an important source of protein, especially for vegetarians. Milk has a huge emotional and cultural connect as well, and is viewed as a comfort food. We use milk in our tea and coffee; we drink it plain; we drink it as lassi and chhaas (buttermilk); we eat it as curd; we freeze it and have ice cream; we clot it and have paneer; and we use it in a large number of sweets that we make. There are a plethora of studies analyzing the effects of milk on various health parameters, but for simplicity's sake, I am presenting you with a take-home message on the subject rather than a detailed study discussion.

If you do not consume milk directly or indirectly as dairy products, you do not need to specifically add it to your diet. Vegetarians might ask, what about protein? There are several non-dairy sources from where a vegetarian or vegan can obtain protein. On the other hand, if like most people you do have a fondness for dairy, I would advise you limit your total consumption to less than half a litre of milk per day. This total includes milk in all its liquid and semi-solid forms such as curd and yogurt.

The next question which comes up is, 'Which type of milk should be consumed?' Most of us have grown up with our milk coming daily to our doorstep, and have never thought of where it comes from. In our household, every morning the Parsi Dairy Farm *doodhwaala* would arrive carrying a large urn of milk on his cycle. The milk would be poured into our home container, kept specifically for the purpose. After the milk was poured he would be handed a pre-paid coupon and the transaction was complete. Even at the pre-dawn hour, the ladies would keep a hawk-eye on the pouring process to prevent any water from diluting the milk.

In later years this was replaced by the plastic pouch, which would be left at the doorstep. Little did we realize that the milk could come from either a buffalo or a cow and that there is a vast difference between the two. Buffalo milk has a significantly higher amount of fat and cholesterol than cow's milk. Twenty years ago, most milk consumed in homes was buffalo milk, but I suspect that this has changed now. A large part of the fat present in milk is saturated fat, which we should aim to keep to a minimum in our diet. This can get converted to cholesterol within the body. The maximum amount of fat is present in buffalo milk, followed by cow milk. The least amount of fat, which is zero, is present in skimmed milk, made from milk powder (and also available in ready cartons). It is also important to note that milk and milk products are the only direct source of cholesterol for vegetarians. If you recollect, cholesterol is only present in foods of animal origin, and milk is of animal origin.

As I mentioned, you should keep your milk consumption to less than half a litre a day. Within this range there may be some who take in only a few teaspoons as part of their tea/coffee, while others consume the entire amount. If your consumption is on the higher side, I would strongly advocate moving towards low-fat milk. For example, if you drink only buffalo milk, I would suggest you shift to cow's milk, and if you drink cow's milk, then make an effort to have skimmed milk. At the end of the day, you need to make the best choice you are comfortable with and can sustain for a long time. There are several of my Punjabi patients for whom drinking skimmed milk is akin to drinking water. For them, I would suggest sticking to the variety they are happy with, but greatly reducing their daily intake.

Antioxidants

Over the last decade, antioxidants have been quite the buzzword in nutrition circles, and have been touted as the cure-all for several chronic diseases. This has led to a very large nutraceutical industry blossoming around them, to the tune of more than 500 million US dollars annually.

If antioxidants are the hero, then free radicals are the villains. Free radicals are chemicals in the body that are formed by various processes during the breakdown of food or due to exposure to tobacco smoke, pollution and radiation. Technically speaking, they are a group of atoms with an uneven number of electrons. In order to get stable they 'steal' an electron from other molecules, which in turn make those molecules unstable. A domino reaction takes place as these molecules carry on stealing an electron from the next one.

You could almost think of it as a reverse game of passing the parcel, where everyone wants to keep the parcel rather than get rid of it. This domino effect creates a wave of damage in all the affected cells, which makes a person prone to heart disease and cancer. Antioxidants confront free radicals and pacify them by giving them an electron to quench their thirst and stabilize them. They are like film heroes who embrace the villains and turn them to the good side, without getting spoiled themselves. The star line-up of antioxidants includes beta carotene (inactive form of vitamin A), vitamin C, vitamin E, lycopene and selenium.

Antioxidant supplements

Unfortunately, most studies on antioxidant supplements have not shown promising results, with some actually showing negative results.

In the early 1990s, there were a number of large studies conducted in which thousands of people were given antioxidants in the form of pills, and followed for several years. It was theorized that antioxidants would ward off the damage done by free radicals and deaths due to heart disease and cancer would be reduced. In fact, these pills were so popular that in our clinic in the US, we used to give all our patients vitamins B, C, and E, along with folic acid. One of the largest studies, titled HOPE (Heart Outcomes Prevention Evaluation), did not live up to its name and dashed all hopes that vitamin E supplementation led to reduction of heart disease. Another large study, called CHAOS (Cambridge Heart Antioxidant Study), lived up to its name and caused chaos in the scientific world. The study did show benefits of vitamin E, but there was debate on the overall results and the authors concluded that, 'The effect of vitamin E treatment on cardiovascular deaths requires further study.' One of the studies on beta carotene supplementation actually showed an increase in lung cancer among smokers.

Eating real food works

The bottom line is that antioxidants do provide benefit against a whole range of diseases, especially heart disease and cancer. However, to gain these benefits there are no short cuts to healthy eating. When antioxidants are consumed in their natural form in foods they contribute towards lowering health risks. Foods rich in antioxidants include:

- *Fruits:* Mangoes, strawberries, raspberries, papaya, plums, cherries, raisins, oranges, peaches, and watermelons.
- *Vegetables:* Tomatoes, broccoli, spinach, red kidney beans (rajma)

Processed foods

Salt was the most vilified food in the 1980s, cholesterol and fat in the 1990s, carbohydrates in the 2000s, and in the current decade that dubious title goes to processed foods. Today, the new fad is to blame processed foods for all that is wrong with our diets, and replace them with 'natural' foods.

The first question we need to answer is what qualifies as processed food. It can be defined as foods that have been altered from their natural states. This is done to extend their shelf life, or for safety reasons, or to improve their palatability. In general, all processed foods are seen as 'bad,' but that is not the case. For example, milk is pasteurised to kill bacteria and make it safer for consumption. This can be considered 'processing' the milk, but in this case it's good for you. Vegetables and fruits often need to be frozen and stored in a particular manner to be able to transport them from farm to plate. This is also a form of processing, but is necessary, and when done correctly, does not diminish the nutritive value. On the other hand, there are several products which are processed in an unhealthy manner, such as bakery items containing trans fats.

Sugar, salt, and different chemicals are often used for processing—carefully reading the nutrition label of packaged foods will inform you if any of these are in the food product. A simple way to identify processed foods are that they usually come packaged in boxes or cans, and are not items which can be made at home from natural ingredients. Common examples are canned soups, ready-to-eat meals, deli meats (such as salami), and sugary breakfast cereals. My suggestion is to limit the amount of these foods in your diet, and eat them only as occasional treats.

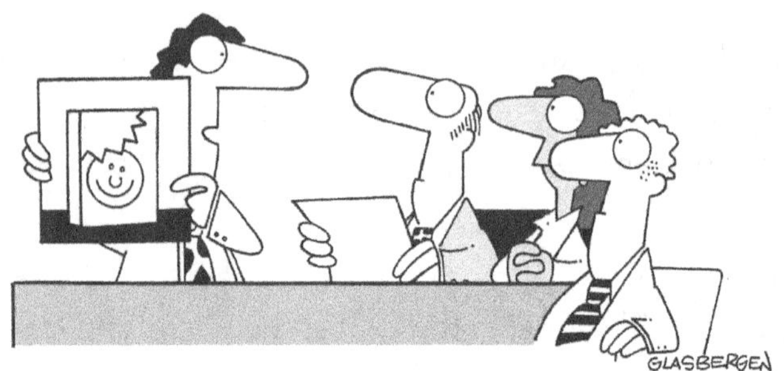

"Our new product has no fat, no cholesterol,
no calories, no sugar, no salt and no preservatives.
The box is empty, but it has exactly what everyone wants!"

Salt

The other day I was watching the movie *Gandhi* (for possibly the twentieth time) when I came across the scene depicting the Dandi march, where the great Mahatma marches to the coastal village of Dandi, and makes salt in defiance of the British salt monopoly. He is arrested a few days later, but the rest of the group carry on to the Dharasana salt factory where they are mercilessly beaten up by the troops, and offer no resistance in return. This was one of the turning points in India's struggle for independence and this scene always brings a tear to my eye (a salty one, I might add). The point behind this rambling introduction is that it always makes me wonder at the irony of our forefathers having fought so hard for the right to make salt, and today for health reasons we need to shun that same salt.

Common salt is chemically known as sodium chloride, and it has been shown that the sodium component has a direct effect on our blood pressure. The recommended intake of salt for everyone, not just those with heart disease, is less than 2,300 mg of sodium a day, which is roughly equal to 6 gm, or a teaspoon of common salt. Please do not confuse the amount of sodium recommended with that of salt. Our daily Indian diet far exceeds that amount, thanks to our habit of putting salt into almost all of our cooking, besides having a partiality to salty food accompaniments, such as papads and pickles. Those with high blood pressure, heart failure, or kidney disease are recommended a lower intake of 1,500 mg of sodium a day. Have a look at the table below to identify commonly-eaten foods which are high in sodium.

Sodium content of sodium-rich foods, per serving

Food item	Serving size	Mg of sodium per serving
Flavouring cubes for soups	1 cube	1,200
Instant tomato soup	1 soup bowl	950
Soya sauce	1 tbsp	933
Processed meat	1 pc / 2 slices	550
Ready-to-use packet masala	1 heaped tsp	540
Soya sauce (low sodium)	1 tbsp	533
Cheddar cheese	1 cube	475
Canned tuna	3 tbsp	336
Chilli sauce	1 tbsp	316
French fries	One medium pack	266
Lime pickles	1 tsp	265
Papad	1 pc	140
Cream and onion chips	1 packet (regular size)	154
Tomato ketchup	1 tbsp	154
Salted chips	1 packet (regular size)	146
Instant noodles	1 small packet	130
Aloo bhujia (namkeen)	1 vati	120
Roasted and salted nuts	15 nuts	46

Spicy food

My friend Garth Spendiff is one of the leading practitioners of Brazilian jujitsu, which is a form of mixed martial arts. He is broad-shouldered, over 6 feet tall, and looks like a person you would not want to mess with. When I was living in the US, we used to run together, followed by dinner. One night at dinner, I saw his face going red and beads of sweat forming around his forehead, which slowly started trickling down the side of his face. I was instantly concerned, and asked him if he was okay. In spite of the redness and sweat he was cheerful, and was clearly enjoying his meal. That's when I realized that it was the Indian spices which were causing this reaction in him. He looked like he was having a heart attack, but in reality was relishing his food, and like Oliver Twist he came back for more.

Most people associate a heart-healthy diet with a bland diet, which may be a reflection of the food served in hospitals. Actually, to be fair to hospital caterers, they need to cater to a wide variety of tastes and palates, and find it safer to keep the food at a lower spice level. Also, patients tend to be on several medications all at once, which—aggravated by spicy food—could potentially give rise to acidity. Indians love their spices, and patients often worry that after being diagnosed with heart disease they are doomed to eating bland food for the rest of their lives. Actually, nothing could be further from the truth. Most spices in their natural forms (as opposed to commercial masala mixes) are heart-friendly and many of them have even been shown to have beneficial properties, especially as antioxidants. Another benefit of adding spices to food is the reduced need to add salt. A word of caution is due here. Spicy food tends to increase acidity in some people, and can aggravate ulcers present in the digestive system. Most heart patients are on blood-thinning medications, which also give rise to some amount of acidity. If you do not suffer from acidity, feel free to add spices to your food and a little bit to your life too.

Your diet guide in a nutshell

Through the chapter, I have tried to present the most scientific data available on nutrition. However, you need to bear in mind that the literature is filled with diets with diametrically opposite recommendations, many of them coming from reputed institutes and doctors. Even as I write this chapter, new research is emerging which questions the role of saturated fat and cholesterol in the development and progression of heart disease. My approach has been to recommend a plan for which there is maximum scientific validation, and has a large body of literature supporting it. Use the five dietary principles I described to guide your food choices. Remember there are no 'poison' foods that you can never eat, nor are there 'wonder' foods that work magically. For long-term success, you need to understand these guidelines, and then design a meal plan which you are comfortable with. Select food from all food groups, but within each one make healthier choices. Both quality and quantity of food matter, and it's important to balance your food intake with your activity in order to achieve and maintain a healthy weight.

Take-home messages

- The diet for heart patients is no different from that recommended for healthy individuals and food should not be cooked separately.

- There can be individual variations in diet, but in general 50-60 per cent calories should come from carbs; 20-30 per cent from fats; and 15-20 per cent from proteins.

- Calories matter. Exercise caloric control to maintain a healthy weight. Divide your daily calories over three main meals and two to three snacks.

- Follow the 1-2-3 rule for your meals: one portion of protein, two portions of grains, and three portions of vegetables.

- Fruits and vegetables should comprise a substantial portion of your daily food intake.

- Complex carbs such as whole grains are recommended, and sugars should be kept to a minimum.

- Cooking oil should be restricted to half a litre per person per month. Saturated fat and cholesterol intake should be kept under control.

- Salt intake should be limited to a teaspoon a day, including salt naturally present in food.

12

Alcohol

(Should you drink to your health?)

MR KISHORE DATE WAS A 60-YEAR-OLD BUSINESSMAN WHO HAD RECENTLY suffered a heart attack. He was sitting across my desk with his wife and daughter, and we were discussing his plan of care. After about half an hour of going through his history and medications, we came to the point where we needed to discuss his lifestyle habits. When I asked him about alcohol consumption, he replied that he was an occasional drinker. Now, if you have been reading the book up to this point, you will know that I have become very wary of the word 'occasional' where it comes to habits, since the word can be used very conveniently to suit the speaker. When I asked him to elaborate how many times a week he drinks, he replied 'Once'. Sitting behind him, his young daughter waved three fingers frantically to correct her dad's version. Mrs Date had no need to be subtle and openly corrected her husband that his idea of once a week was really three times a week. A friendly family debate ensued, and I can safely say that I have witnessed hundreds of these debates, some of which are not very friendly.

Whenever I have lectured a group of patients and their families on the subject of heart disease, the women are invariably more interested than the men in most aspects of the talk. When the topic shifts to lifestyle changes, exercise and nutrition, you can see the men sink a little lower in their seat while the women seem to get even more attentive. But the moment the subject of alcohol comes up, suddenly the men are wide awake, smiling. The look on their face seems to say, 'You have burdened us with all these strict dos and don'ts and life is going to be so hard now, with our wives having even more control, but now you are talking our subject. We know that alcohol is good for the heart and is our one final refuge in this otherwise bleak future.'

Of course, all men do not drink and feel the same way, but I am sure you get the picture. The media loves a good story, and anything on alcohol makes for one. Whenever there is any study showing the good effects of things that are traditionally thought of as 'bad for health', they get more airtime. A study showing that alcohol or chocolate is good for your heart gets much more coverage than one showing that spinach or broccoli is good for your heart.

Is alcohol good or bad for your heart?

The French have a much lower rate of heart disease than the Americans, even though their fat consumption is the same. This led to the coining of the term 'French Paradox'. Researchers have thought that the consumption of red wine may be one of the reasons for this phenomenon, and hence red wine has been the subject of maximum focus. It should also be noted that many of the studies have been sponsored by the wine industry in different parts of the world. The bulk of the evidence shows that when alcohol is consumed in moderation, it does have a beneficial effect on heart disease. However, before you take this sentence too literally, there are many clarifications which need to be made, the most important being that of the word 'moderation'.

In most areas of food consumption, especially soft drinks, the Indian version of large is probably half the size of the American version. At 7-Eleven stores in the US, a 'Big Gulp' beverage is about two litres, which is equal to seven cans of Coca Cola. And this is meant for one person! But in one area, the Indian version of large beats the American, and that is the size of a peg of alcohol. In India, one drink is 60 ml of liquor (such as whisky or vodka), while in America it's 45 ml. In alcohol content, 45 ml of liquor is equivalent to 150 ml of wine or 330 ml of beer. In the studies that have been conducted, moderate drinking is considered to be (up to) two drinks a day for men and one drink a day for women.

One always needs to be cautious by patients' definitions, especially when it comes to alcohol. The other day I met Mr Jayesh Rupani, the 48-year-old I mentioned earlier, who told me that after bypass surgery the only problem he faced was that he could not control his laughter. Clearly, Jayesh was a jovial gentleman who lived life large (literally too, he was 114 kg). Since he was a restaurateur and nightclub owner, I was worried that alcohol consumption could be an 'occupational hazard', and questioned him about it. He assured me that he just had one large drink a day. It turned out that he lived large in this aspect too, and considered a peg to be 75 ml. Now, that is large even by Patiala standards!

The other clarification that needs to be made is that while moderate drinking has shown to reduce heart disease, this is in specific reference to coronary heart disease. When taken in excess though, alcohol can lead to cardiomyopathy (swelling of the heart), and abnormal heart rhythms. Besides these, excessive alcohol may also lead to liver disease and has been recently implicated in some forms of cancer.

How does it work?

The beneficial effects of alcohol have been thought to be through raising good cholesterol (HDL), as well as through antioxidant properties. A lot of these antioxidant properties are obtained from the skin of the grape, which has a substance called resveratrol. The debate is whether the beneficial effects of wine are only because of the grapes, or whether there is some 'special property' that wine possesses aside from the grapes. If it's only the grapes, then drinking grape juice could have the same beneficial effects, much to the happiness of many of my patients' wives.

Besides these effects, alcohol is also theorized to reduce the clotting property of blood in the arteries, having a mini-aspirin effect.

Which alcohol is best for you?

As I had mentioned earlier, the maximum research has been around wine, especially red wine. However, there are studies which show that other forms of alcohol have similar effects too. I suggest that if you drink in moderation, select the alcohol of your choice. If you like all equally, then opt for red wine.

So, should I drink or not?

My advice on this is very clear. If you do not drink currently, please do not start drinking with the idea that it's good for your heart. However, if you do enjoy a drink, then do so in moderation. I would personally define moderation as a maximum of one or two drinks, three days per week. A lot of my patients ask if they do not drink Monday to Friday, could they have six drinks on Saturday night. The answer to that is clearly no, and also, just to remind you, one drink is 45 ml of liquor.

Another common question is when can a person start drinking after a heart attack or interventional procedure. I would personally suggest waiting for a period of at least four weeks after the event.

I hope this clarifies the topic of alcohol. I also hope that by the time you have reached this point in the book, you have imbibed all the other heart-healthy tips I have been writing about and not just imbibed (pun intended) the part on alcohol. A lot of patients will sit through a long consult, during which we discuss all the changes they need to make. When they go home and their spouse asks them what the doctor said, their only reply is, 'He said it's okay for me to drink.'

Let me end with my favourite alcohol and heart disease story. My entire staff and I were at one of our colleague's wedding reception at the Taj President Hotel in Mumbai, with many cardiologists in attendance. A lot of our patients were there too, including one of our oldest and dearest, Rusi Vimadalal. If you recollect, I had introduced Rusi to you in the chapter on nutrition, when he had complained that he did not want to eat only *'ghaas-foos'*. Rusi had his angioplasty in 2003 and has been following up in our risk reduction program ever since and progressing well. During the function, Rusi sidled up to me and very secretly pulled out something from his pocket. When he opened his hand I was shocked to see a miniature bottle of Johnny Walker Black Label whisky in his palm. He told me that he suspected the function would be 'dry' and true to his boy scout's motto of 'always be prepared', he did not leave home without his trusty companion. And to think I tell people never to leave home without a pedometer!

Take-home messages

- Studies have shown that alcohol in moderation can be beneficial for the heart, but when taken in excess can cause harm.

- If you don't drink, do not start with the idea of gaining benefits for the heart. If you do drink, do so in moderation.

- Moderation can be defined as two drinks for men, and one for women. One drink is 45 ml of hard liquor, or 330 ml of beer, or 150 ml of wine.

13

Weight Loss
(What works and what doesn't)

THE FIRST TIME I MET ARVIND GURJAR, HE HAD TO BE DRAGGED INTO my office. Well, not literally, since he was 152 kg, but he did need to be coaxed by his father to enrol into our preventive cardiology program. Arvind was 25 years old, and his father was extremely concerned since there was a family history of heart disease, and he certainly seemed to be headed down the wrong path. Clearly his father wanted him to lose weight, but I was not sure whether Arvind felt the same way. So I asked to meet with him separately. I often find that the information you learn from a patient without their family members present is very different. When I met him alone, I sensed that he did want to lose weight (most people at 152 kg would), but he did not want it as much as his parents wanted it for him. It took almost a month of working with him to finally get him well and truly motivated to lead a healthier lifestyle for himself and not for anyone else.

We set a six-month target of 10 per cent weight loss, to be achieved through a negative caloric balance of 500 calories per day. After six months he had lost about 6 kg, which was less than his target, but encouraged him to stick with the program. In another three months, he had lost a total of 10 kg, and seemed very excited when I met him one morning. He said, 'Doc, for the first time in years I was able to get into a pair of jeans,' and this meant more to him than what the weighing scale showed. I am happy to tell you that Arvind is now 111 kg, in a span of 15 months, and is all set to break the two-figure barrier in the near future. What is more important is that he did it the sensible way, which is also the hard way.

In this chapter, we will talk more about the right way to lose weight, but before we do that, you need to figure out whether you need to lose weight in the first place. And if yes, how much.

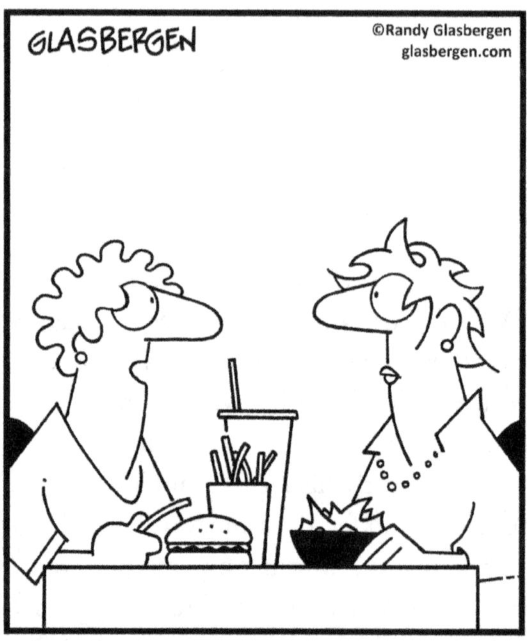

"My doctor wants me to reach a normal weight. But if everyone is heavy now, then *overweight is the new normal!*"

How much weight do I need to lose?

You need to first calculate your body mass index (BMI) to check whether you fall in the normal, overweight or obese category. Refer to Chapter 4 for the Easy BMI Calculator.

Normal weight

If your BMI is less than 25 kg/m², then by the World Health Organization (WHO) standards, you fall in the normal weight category. However, there are several medical organizations which suggest that, for Indians, the BMI cut-off for normal weight should be 23 kg/m². This is because Indians tend to have a higher percentage of body fat compared to Westerners at the same BMI. If your BMI is between 23–25 kg/m², I would suggest a modest weight loss of a few kilos, but would not be overly concerned. However, if you belong to the category of individuals who have a thin frame and a large potbelly, then I would definitely recommend some weight loss.

Overweight

You are categorized overweight if your BMI falls between 25 and 30 kg/m². In my experience, a majority of patients tend to fall into this category, and can be described by that age-old title of 'pleasantly plump', or as most Indians would say, 'healthy'. As I had said in an earlier chapter, all you need to do is stand at the entrance of a city mall on a Sunday and observe the size of people as they enter. Most of them will be in the overweight category. If you read our health and glamour magazines, you will get the impression that as a country we have become obsessed with slimming, both for cosmetic and for health reasons. Somehow, that's not the sense I get in my medical practice. On a weekly basis, I will come across a patient and his family who are concerned about his loss of weight after surgery. What's interesting is that, in most cases, the person has lost some weight, but is still fairly overweight. They get rather startled (and a bit annoyed, I suspect) when I react to their concern by saying that it's good the person has lost weight, and that he should actually lose some more. I have rarely had my patients' family members come up to me and say that they want their patient to lose weight (unless they are grossly overweight). We face a great cultural battle when it comes to weight loss. For centuries, being overweight in India has been looked upon as a sign of prosperity, and a person is considered to be from a '*khata peeta*' family if they tip the scale at numbers higher than the WHO would like. Therefore, in spite of this seemingly modern trend towards slimness as popularized by the new Bollywood look, most Indians are happy with having their 'prosperity' show.

I was reminded of this again when I met Rohit Pawar in my clinic. He is a 43-year-old senior manager with UTI, and looked very trim. He was 5 feet, 8 inches tall, and weighed 65.3 kg. All his reports were perfect, but he seemed very worried. The cause of his worry was that he had lost 5 kg, and everyone around him was very concerned. My first question was whether he had done anything to cause the weight loss, and he said he had started walking every day for exercise. This clearly explained his weight loss and I was perplexed by the worry. Here was someone who was exercising, feeling good, and his blood parameters had improved, and his family was worried that he had lost weight! He had actually stopped walking because of it. I assured him that he was perfectly healthy and should resume his exercise, but this episode cemented my belief that most Indians like their family looking 'healthy'.

To get back to the original point: if your BMI is between 25 and 30 kg/m², then you should attempt to lose 10 per cent of your body weight over the next six months, with the weight loss divided evenly over this period of time.

Obese

Though we tend to use the phrase overweight and obese interchangeably, there are precise definitions for both terms. A person is considered obese if the BMI is 30 kg/m² or more. To make it easier to visualize, a person who is 5 feet 7 inches tall and weighs 87 kg, has a BMI of 30 kg/m². If you do fall into this category, then your risk for several diseases, including heart disease, diabetes, stroke and cancer, greatly increases. A good starting point would be to lose 10 per cent of your weight over 6 months. Using the above example, you would need to reduce 9 kg (10 per cent of 87 kg) over 6 months, or 1.5 kg per month. Once you achieve it, your next goal should be to strive for a BMI of 25, which for a 5 feet 7 inches person would be 72 kg. You should set a target to get to this weight over the next 6 to 12 months. Thus, in little over a year, it is possible to move from obese to normal weight.

Of course, this is often easier said than done—but with a sensible plan, it is eminently achievable.

RECOMMENDED WEIGHT LOSS

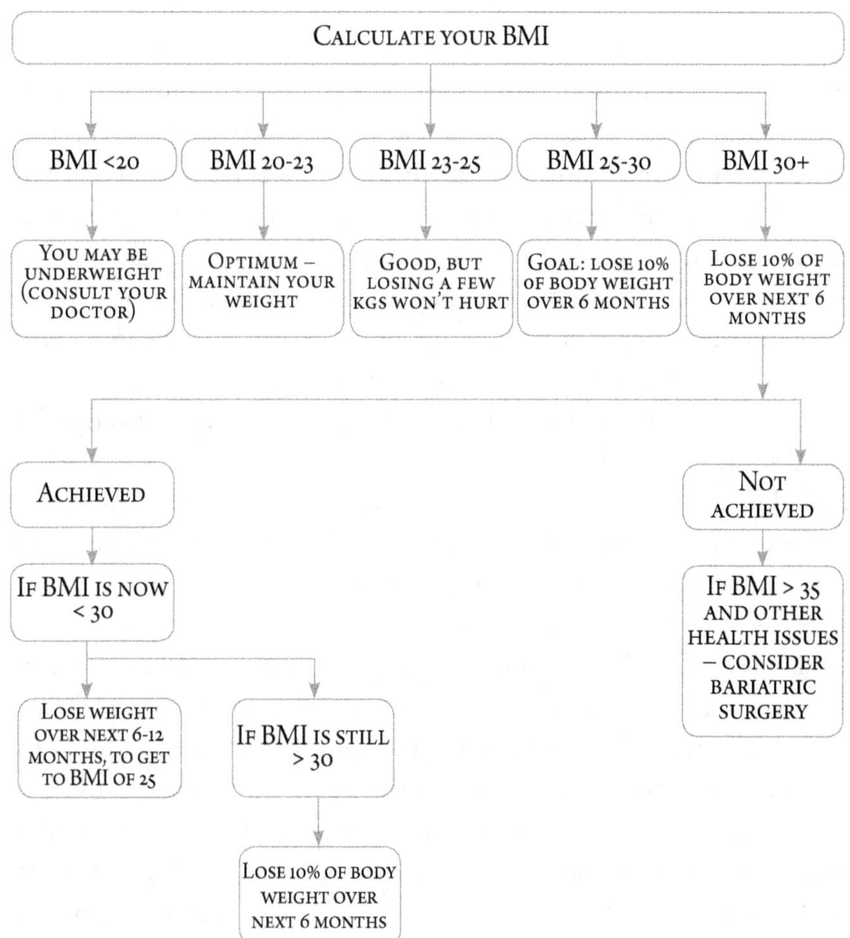

What works for weight loss?

One night we were having dinner with the parents of my daughter's friends. The conversation strayed in the direction of weight loss (after the usual grumbling of the amount of homework kids get, and the travails of finding a good maid). Weight loss is a subject on which everyone has an opinion, and often a strong one. I find these discussions very amusing and was being a quiet listener when my opinion was sought. I told them that after many years of experience and study, I had finally found the secret for sure-fire success. By this time, I could see that the men were interested too. I paused for a bit and then leaned forward and told them that there were two steps to success: eat less and exercise more. I was only stating the obvious, and did not expect them to take it seriously. I was pleasantly surprised when my daughter returned from school one day and said that a friend of hers had told her, 'Your daddy said that if you want to lose weight you need to exercise more and eat less.' Clearly, some of them had taken the advice to heart that night.

Actually, it all boils down to simple math.

Change in weight = calories in − calories out

At a basic level, this equation is fundamentally true. If you consume more calories than you burn, you will gain weight, and if you burn more calories than you consume, you will lose weight. Of course, there are other factors, such as metabolism, which come into play, but at the end of it, this simple math largely holds good. I'd like to point out that if you are looking at calories purely from the angle of weight loss, then it's only a numbers game. But from a health perspective, the quality of food that you consume is extremely important. In other words, it is possible to eat very little of unhealthy food and lose weight, and it is possible to eat healthy food in a larger quantity and put on weight. Clearly the best option is to consume the right food in the right amount.

'Calories in' come through only one source, which is the food you eat. 'Calories out' come from three different sources:

- *Basal metabolic rate*: The build-up and breakdown of energy is known as metabolism, which is a continuous process in your body and burns calories. This goes on unconsciously all day in your body, and is the bulk of your daily caloric consumption, forming about 70 per cent of the total.

- *Thermic effect of feeding*: Believe it or not, you actually burn calories while digesting the food you have eaten. This forms close to 10 per cent of daily caloric expenditure.
- *Physical activity:* this forms about 20 per cent of your daily caloric expenditure, and is really the only variable which is completely in your control and you need to make an effort to maximize it.

Create a calorie deficit

If you want to lose weight it's essential to create a calorie deficit, which is the difference between the calories you consume, and those you burn. A sensible deficit would be about 500 calories a day through diet and physical activity. This can be achieved by eating about 300 calories a day less than your usual diet (cutting back on one soft drink, and two slices of bread could achieve that), and by increasing your physical activity to burn 200 calories extra, which is equivalent to half an hour of brisk walking. A deficit of 500 calories a day would lead to a 3,500 calorie loss in a week, which is roughly equivalent to half a kg of fat loss. If you can sustain this for a month, you could lose 2 kg, which is great, especially if you can maintain this over time. Unfortunately though, the human body is not a machine, and while this formula generally holds true, there are several variables which could alter the actual weight lost. If you are obese to begin with, you could create a larger calorie deficit, even up to 1,000 calories a day. For that you would need to further reduce your food intake, but as a general rule, do not consume less than 1,200 calories a day as part of your daily diet.

Count your calories in and out

In my experience, one of the simplest and best tools to aid in weight loss is maintaining a daily record of the food you consume, and the exercise you do. You could do it in a low-tech manner like I do, which is a simple handwritten diary, or you could use one of the several hundred free applications available today on your smart phone. Most of these applications will calculate the calories you have consumed through your food, as well as those burned through exercise. Trust me, if you are able to maintain this for an extended period of time, you will gain success. Just the act of recording your diet daily brings about a sense of awareness, which will lead to change over time. It's also a good idea to record your weight on a regular basis—I would suggest once a week. From now on, your diary, along with your pedometer, will be your conscience!

Exercise and weight loss

One of the main reasons people exercise is to lose weight. They figure that, through exercise, they will be able to burn a lot of calories, which will lead to weight loss. I am a great fan of exercise, so it pains me to break the bad news to you: exercise has many wonderful effects, but it's not as great a calorie-burner as we think it to be, or would like it to be. Make no mistake, exercise does burn calories, but just not as much as we think it does. On an average, walking one mile (which is 1.6 km) burns 100 calories for a person of average weight. At this point, suffice it to say, that where weight is concerned, your diet probably plays a greater role in weight loss than exercise alone, though a combination is the best.

A few years ago, some friends of mine took up walking in order to lose weight. They would walk an entire round of the Mahalaxmi Race Course in Mumbai, which is fairly big, about 2.4 km. They would then go across to the Willingdon Club and have a large glass of fresh orange juice. The famous Chowpatty Beach juice stall, Bachelorr's, had just opened their outlet at the club, and my friends felt that they had earned their treat. They were perplexed when, after a month of exercise, they did not see their weight dropping. I sat down with them and burst their bubble. Their walk probably burned off 150 calories, after which they treated themselves to orange juice, which was made up of three to four oranges and a spoonful of sugar, and was about 200 calories. The net effect of their 'healthy' evening out was a 50-calorie weight gain!

Before this puts you off exercise, I must hasten to add that the benefits of exercise should definitely not be viewed through the narrow prism of weight loss alone. It's just to caution you from falling into a false sense of comfort. The good news is that, if you exercise vigorously, for the next several hours after you finish your session, your metabolism will be a slight bit higher and you will continue burning extra calories.

Also, while research has shown that in your initial weight loss efforts, diet probably plays a greater role than exercise, in weight maintenance they have nearly equal roles. The table below shows the amount of calories you burn in an hour for various types of exercise.

Activity	Calories burned in an hour for a person weighing 70 kg
Cycling (19-22 km/h)	560
Stationary cycling	420
Walking (5-6 km/h)	300
Jogging (8-9 km/h)	560
Aerobic dancing	420
Badminton (non-competitive)	315
Tennis (doubles)	420
Swimming (freestyle)	560
Squash	840
Sitting still	63

Does exercise at low intensity burn more fat than high-intensity exercise?

The body primarily uses fats and carbohydrates as sources of energy. These are supplied from the food we eat. At rest and low-intensity exercise, about 60 per cent of energy is derived from fat, and the remainder from carbohydrate. As exercise intensity increases from mild to moderate to hard, the relative contribution of fat declines while that of carbohydrate increases. Although the relative amount of fat burned decreases, the absolute amount may remain the same (or even increase), since at higher intensity the overall caloric expenditure increases.

Example: If low-intensity exercise burns 100 calories in 30 minutes, and the contribution from fat is 60 per cent (note: contribution from fat is never

100 per cent), then you will burn 60 calories of fat during that half hour. However, if you exercise at a higher intensity, the contribution from fat may decrease to 35 per cent, but the overall calories burned may increase to 200. Therefore, absolute fat calories burned will be 70, higher than those burned at a low intensity, though the relative contribution has decreased.

As mentioned above, the good effects of an exercise bout last for a long time after the bout is over, and you continue to burn calories at a slightly elevated rate for a while. In fact, the harder you exercise, the more fat calories you will burn during the recovery period. Your metabolic rate may be increased for a period of 24 hours after a bout of exercise. Therefore, there is added weight loss benefit with higher intensity exercise. However, it is important to remember that there is an inverse relationship between intensity and time. If you exercise at a higher intensity, you will be able to exercise for a shorter time. There is no magic formula to figure out the best combination, but a practical approach is to exercise at an intensity that allows you to complete 30–60 minutes of the exercise comfortably.

Don't forget physical activity

The 'secret' formula I shared with you spoke about eating less and exercising more, but there is a third component too—increasing physical activity. As explained earlier in the book, physical activity and exercise are similar, but not the same. Often, when we try to lose weight, our focus is on structured exercise, and we forget to increase daily physical activity such as climbing stairs and parking the car further away. These seem to be inconsequential by themselves, but when done repeatedly over a prolonged period of time, yield great results. Let me give you a simple example.

Mr Ganesh Rao lives in Kandivli and works in south Mumbai, so needs to take the local train daily. Luckily for him, his house is only half a kilometre from the station and it takes him five to six minutes in the morning to walk to the station and the same time back in the evening. Last year, he got a promotion and to celebrate, bought himself a motorcycle. He now rides the bike to the station and parks it there. Let's take a look at the consequences of this small action on his weight. An average person burns about 65 calories, when they walk a kilometre, which is what Mr Rao did to and from the station daily. Assuming he did this 300 times a year, he would burn close to 20,000 calories, which is about 3 kg of weight. In other words, all else remaining equal in his life, Mr Rao would put on 3 kg of weight in a year just because he stopped his daily five-minute walk to the station. Similarly, think of how many 'small' walks you could do in your daily life which could help you shed off those unwanted pounds.

Get fidgety

First, the world of medicine looked at the benefits of exercise, then it looked at the benefits of being physically active, and now the latest research is on the benefits of movement—any movement. Or, to be more precise, research is looking at the ill-effects of being sedentary. A number of different studies done in the past few years have found that for every additional hour a day you spend sitting, you increase your risk for a number of chronic health conditions. In fact, one large study done in Australia found that for every additional hour of television watched per day, your risk of dying increased by 11 per cent! I am not suggesting that you don't watch television, but the moral of the story is that you need to decrease the total amount of time a day you spend sitting. Researchers at the Mayo Clinic actually showed this by making a group of people wear underwear with motion sensors on them to detect every single movement. They found that those people who were heavy tended to sit more, while the lean ones were more restless and spent two more hours a day on their feet (not exercising, but just moving around). They even coined a term for this type of calorie burning—NEAT, which stands for non-exercise activity thermogenesis. Think of all the people around you whom you would describe as 'fidgety'—the kind who just can't stand still. It's not a coincidence that most of them will be thin.

Beware of binges

Almost anyone on a diet program will tell you that they are very disciplined throughout the week with their diet and exercise, but allow themselves to 'let loose' over the weekend. While this sounds sensible, it will greatly slow down or even halt your progress towards weight loss.

Let's assume that you have embarked on a healthy eating and exercise regimen over the past few months, and you walk for an hour, five days a week, at a speed of 5 km/hour. So, in total you are walking 25 km per week as exercise. Thanks to this regime you have lost about 3 kg of weight and are now 'weight stable'. In other words, your intake is equal to your output. You are pleased with yourself and decide that you are allowed to let go or 'cheat' once a week. On Saturday nights you allow yourself to indulge in a few cocktails, unlimited starters, followed by a nice heavy dinner, washed down with some dessert. During the course of the evening and night, it would not be difficult to consume about 1,500-1,800 calories, which would be about 1,000 calories in excess over your normal dinner. Remember, you burn 100 calories for every mile (1.6 km) walked. Therefore, you would need to walk 16 km extra the next week just to repent for the sins of Saturday night. So now you need to walk 41 km during the next week, just to maintain your weight (your usual 25 plus 16 extra). Assuming you manage to do that over the next six days, you are then back to square one for the week. Now it's Saturday again, and time for your once-a-week treat, which will take you the next six days to get rid of. Do you get the picture? And this example assumes that you will burn off the extra calories. If you don't, then instead of weight loss, you will gain weight!

The moral of the story is that you can certainly loosen up once a week, but just by very little. You have got to be careful about bingeing, since that just won't work from a weight loss perspective.

Be consistent

Without doubt, the resolve to 'lose weight this year' is the most popular resolution made on January 1 each year. And without doubt it's the most commonly broken resolution by January 31 of each year. Losing weight and keeping it off is very difficult. Consistency is the key for long-term success. You need to find creative ways by which you can regulate your food intake and increase physical activity. Make rules for yourself which you know you can follow for the rest of your life. And at the end of the day, remember that following a healthy lifestyle is more important than just weight loss. You may not lose all the weight you want to, but as long as you eat right and exercise you will continue to get health benefits.

Take-home messages

- If you are overweight, you should aim to lose 10 per cent of your weight over a 6-month period. If you are obese (BMI > 30), after you lose the initial 10 per cent, you should aim to achieve a BMI of 25 over the next 6-12 months.

- Change in weight = calories in − calories out. If you consume more calories than you burn you will put on weight, and vice versa.

- A sensible weight loss plan involves creating a 500-calorie daily deficit through a combination of diet and exercise. However, make sure you consume at least 1,200 calories per day while dieting.

- Exercise has many wonderful health effects, but is not a great calorie burner. It's important to increase daily physical activity as well.

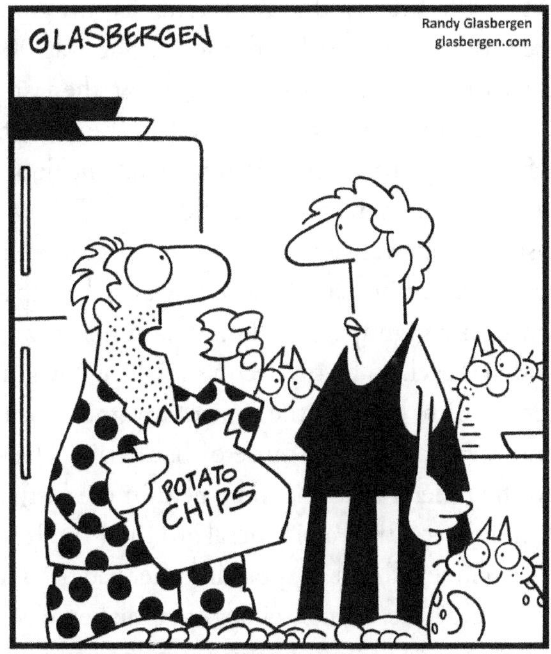

"My diet says I can have 1800 calories per day. It doesn't say anything about NIGHT!"

14

Stress Management

(Unloading your heart)

Throughout the book I have shared real life examples of patients to better explain the mechanism of heart disease and steps towards its prevention. Now, I would like to share a very personal experience with you.

On January 5, 2006, I received the sad news that my grand-aunt Daulat Wadia had passed away in the early afternoon. She was 90 years old and had led a full life, though she had been ailing for the last few years. She was my grandfather's brother's wife, and lived in the same building as my grandparents. My grandmother, Freny Wadia, lived one floor above her, and they had been the best of friends for over 50 years. This was one '*jethani-derrani*' relationship which was very warm, and they grew even closer to each other after their respective husbands passed away. I had spent a large part of my childhood in my grandparents' home, and hence was close to both ladies, and considered each to be my second mother. My grandmother was in reasonably good health, but—at the time of my grand-aunt's death—had been homebound for a few days because of back pain. She was, therefore, unable to attend the funeral that was to be held in the early evening.

Our entire family was at the Parsi funeral ground (The Towers of Silence), when we received a phone call that my grandmother had become unconscious. We rushed home to find her semi-conscious and took her to Bombay Hospital at once. At the hospital, a CT scan of the brain showed that she had had a massive haemorrhagic (bleeding) stroke, and she passed away in a few hours. She was very close to my heart, and to this day I wonder if things would have been different had one of us been by her side and not gone to the funeral. I have no doubt in my mind that the loss of her companion of more than 50 years caused the sudden stroke. She was remarkably healthy for an 87-year-old lady, and it's hard for me to believe that it was mere coincidence. There is certainly a strong mind-body connection, which medical science has not fully understood yet, but we are learning more each day. Since ancient times the heart has been considered the seat of emotions, but it's only in the recent past that we have a better understanding of how exactly our mind and our emotions affect our heart.

The InterHeart Study, which looked at 26,000 people who had a heart attack across 52 countries, showed that psychosocial factors were one of the 9 most important causes of heart disease. 'Psychosocial factors' is an umbrella term which includes stress, depression, anger, hostility, and social isolation. The presence of any of these can increase your chances of heart disease by two to three-folds.

What is stress?

In medical terms, stress has been defined as the non-specific response of the body to any demand for change. As you can see, the definition is as vague as our understanding of the term. Stress sharpened pre-historic man's fight-or-flight response. Confronted with any stressful situation, he had to decide to fight or take flight. So, if he saw another man courting the woman of his dreams, he would stand up and fight. But if he stumbled upon a lion in the jungle, who was with the lioness of his dreams, he would likely turn and run as fast as he possibly could. To aid him in his escape, his body would secrete certain hormones. These would speed up his heart rate and allow more blood flow to his muscles. In the concrete jungle we live in today, we are unlikely to come across a lion (though we do have political 'tigers'), but if the Sensex fell by 500 points in a day, then the response would pretty much be the same. If you are an investor, your heart rate would shoot through the roof, your sweat glands would be overactive, and your chest would start hurting. These responses are modulated by a part of your nervous system called the sympathetic nervous system, which releases the hormone adrenaline. Often while watching a sporting event you would have heard the commentator say that the athlete's adrenaline is pumping.

Stress cannot be measured

Stress is the only cardiac risk factor that cannot be measured. I can tell you that your BP is 130/80, or that your cholesterol is 220 mg/dl, but I cannot put a number to your stress. Since we cannot measure stress, it becomes hard to define it in an individual. After all, stress is a normal part of life, which when present in the right amount helps us function optimally. It's only when stress becomes excessive does it turn to distress.

How does stress affect the heart and body

Stress is an independent or direct risk factor for heart disease, but it also acts indirectly via its influence on other risk factors, such as high blood pressure, cholesterol and obesity. For example, individuals who are highly stressed may have wrong eating habits and not exercise, which will increase their risk. In this case, stress has an indirect effect on the heart.

Stress can directly influence the heart through the nervous system. Due to stress, the hormone adrenaline is released which causes the heart to beat faster, and at the same time leads to narrowing of the coronary arteries. Your blood pressure and breathing rate also increases. In addition, it leads to an increase in sweating, slowing down of digestive activity, and narrowing of blood vessels in different parts of the body. All of these responses are designed to help you fight or take flight. These are protective in the short term, but when present for several years, they tend to have negative effects on the body. It's like having an emergency system that is on alert mode all the time.

There are several different manifestations of chronic stress—which may be physical or mental—on the body. The physical signs of chronic stress include frequent headaches, fatigue, backache, sweaty palms, fast heart beat, sleep problems, and stomach problems such as acidity, and irritable bowel syndrome. Stress also affects the immune system, making you more prone to infections, and can aggravate skin conditions such as acne, psoriasis and eczema.

The effects of chronic stress on the mind affect our mood and emotions, which ultimately affect our behaviour. It may lead to anger and irritability on the one end, and sadness and depression on the other. Anxiety, decrease in concentration, and loss of memory are also side effects of chronic stress.

What are stressors?

Stressors are anything that can make you stressed. Stressors can be divided into major and minor, though you need to remember that this is not a foolproof classification. Someone may consider a delayed flight a minor stressor, while another might consider it major.

Here is a list of minor stressors that usually take place in daily life. By no means is it a complete list.

- Job stress
- Minor illness
- Daily commute
- Inflation
- Weather

Very often, if minor stressors persist for a while, they can turn into major stressors. On the other hand, some situations in life clearly qualify as major, and here is a list of some of them:

- Serious illness or death in the family
- Loss of job
- Relationship issues
- Divorce
- Financial constraints

Responses to stressors

I think we need to distinguish between stress as a noun and stress as a verb. I don't think my ninth grade English grammar teacher, the late great Mr Joe Sheth, would approve of this classification, but here is the way I look at it. A noun is a name, place, animal or thing. By that logic, stress should be a noun, since it's a 'thing' which when present affects us. On the other hand, a verb is 'an action', and our reaction to stress is an 'action'. In my opinion, the verb part of the stress equation is far more important, and is something we need to channel into positive energy rather than negative.

I believe one way to do this is through our attitude. I once came across a lovely lesson on attitude in the strangest of places—the washroom of a restaurant! While living in the US, I was eating at Hyman's, a famous restaurant in Charleston. At the end of the meal, I had to use the washroom. Next to the door was a small folder with leaflets, which the customers were encouraged to take. It was on the subject of attitude, written by the American author Charles Swindoll. The words are so profound, I still have that leaflet which I picked up that day in 1998.

Attitude – by Charles Swindoll

The longer I live, the more I realize the impact of attitude on life. Attitude, to me, is more important than facts. It is more important than the past, than education, than money, than circumstances, than failures, than successes, than what other people think or say or do.
The remarkable thing is we have a choice every day regarding the attitude we will embrace for that day. We cannot change our past...we cannot change the fact that people will act in a certain way. We cannot change the inevitable. The only thing we can do is play on the one string we have, and that is our attitude.... I am convinced that life is 10 per cent what happens to me and 90 per cent how I react to it.
And so it is with you...we are in charge of our attitudes.

I truly believe that we are in charge of our attitudes, which directly affect our responses to stressors. In the times we live in today, there are going to be numerous stressors in our daily life, but our reaction to them is largely in our control. Let's look at the example of traffic. If you live in any big city in India today, rush-hour traffic in the evening can be a nightmare, especially with everyone turning into Formula One drivers in narrow, crowded lanes. We have this unique ability to create a gridlock in seconds. As a driver, you have two options. Like most people, you can get agitated and every now and then roll down your window and shout abuses at the other drivers. Or, you can choose to be calm, turn up your radio a little louder and sit through the moment, realizing that there is nothing you can directly do about the traffic, but you can control your reaction.

Dealing with stress

Chirag Mehta was a young entrepreneur who had just made his first million (dollars, of course) by selling a stake in his IT gaming company. He had come with his whole family to meet me for his father, who had suffered a heart attack. Chirag looked at least 20 kg overweight, and considering his father had had an attack at 54, I knew that he already had two risk factors for heart disease.

As is often the case, after finishing his father's consult, the family asked me to talk some sense into young Chirag, since he ate junk food, did not exercise, and was always stressed out. To complete his risk-factor profile, I asked him whether he smoked and he promptly said he didn't. At the end of the consult, as the family left my room, Chirag lingered back (as is also often the case) and told me in a hushed tone that he smoked a pack a day, but his family did not know it. I often wonder why fully-grown men need to hide from the family the fact that they smoke. I guess one advantage from a health point of view is that if they are hiding and smoking, then the overall consumption is probably less than what it might have been if it was out in the open.

When I told Chirag that smoking was the single worst thing he could do for his health, he said that he was so stressed that he had to smoke. According to him, smoking relieved his stress and allowed him to cope. I have heard this excuse from smokers several times before and it would be funny if the consequences were not so grave. When you smoke, your heart rate momentarily increases and your blood vessels narrow, increasing your pressure. So, if anything, smoking actually has the opposite effect of calming you down. In fact, in a very interesting study done in the UK, researchers found that smoking actually caused anxiety. Chain smokers had such a dependence on nicotine that they felt irritable and stressed in between cigarettes. Smoking the next cigarette helped relieve this stress, which ironically was due to smoking in the first place. After quitting and getting over the initial withdrawal symptoms, smokers actually experience a drop in their stress levels.

Stress management techniques

Now that we have confirmed that smoking is not a stress buster, let's try to explore some real solutions for stress reduction. When tackling any problem, the first step is to identify and accept there is a problem. In my opinion, almost all of us living in the 21st century have a degree of stress in our lives, whether we accept it or not. The various stress management techniques I will be talking about will be applicable to you and will help even if you feel that you are not stressed.

Meditation

The first time in my life I was introduced to meditation was, strangely enough, in California. I say strangely, since India is considered the world capital of meditation, and I should have had this experience at home rather than in a foreign country. This was in 1997, and I was doing a short internship under Dr Dean Ornish at his Preventive Medicine and Research Institute in California. Dr Ornish is a pioneer of preventive cardiology, and was instrumental in coining the phrase, 'reversal of heart disease'. Yoga and meditation were integral components of his teaching, and my meditation experience was as part of the program.

I had heard people talk about how difficult it can be to truly meditate and keep your mind clear of thought, and personally I found that hard to understand. I mean, how difficult could it be to think of nothing, right? During the session, the teacher told us that our mind is like a monkey and we need to try and make it stand still. She guided us through a series of steps and then asked us to think of nothing for the next five minutes. What I had thought to be easy was actually turning out to be close to impossible. Try as I might, the monkey would jump around and never remain still. I think the longest 'thought-free' spell I managed must have been 15 seconds! However, after doing it for a few sessions, it did get easier, and I began to look forward to it as part of my daily routine.

There are several different meditation techniques, and since I am not an expert on the subject, I will not attempt to create one more. However, there are certain aspects which are common to most of these techniques that you should incorporate in your meditation practice.

- The most essential of these is finding a quiet space to meditate in. I am sure enlightened souls can meditate even in the middle of 30 million people (like they do at the Kumbh Mela), but since most of us are not enlightened, let us start with a quiet space.
- The next step is to make sure you are comfortable. The yogic posture of padmasana, or the lotus pose, is very conducive to meditation, but if you find that difficult, it's okay to be seated in any comfortable position, on the ground or on a chair.
- Spend the first few minutes focusing on your breath and gradually try to clear your mind of all other thoughts. There are different techniques to help you focus: try a few and decide which works best for you. You can chant a specific mantra or word such as 'Om', and repeat it in your mind. Another method is guided imagery where you visualize yourself in a location which is soothing, or focus your mind on a specific vision, such as a distant sunset. Your thoughts will be distracted at first, but as you practice, you will be able to achieve a state of mindfulness, with greater ease.
- There is no specific duration for which the meditation needs to last, but I would recommend 10-15 minutes daily.

Prayer can also be considered a form of meditation, and lately, there has been much scientific interest in the power of prayers to heal. Since time immemorial human beings have turned to prayer in times of trouble. This reminds me of one of the famous couplets of the renowned poet-saint Kabir, which loosely translates as follows: *In sorrowful times, we all pray; in joyful times no one prays. If we were to pray in joyful times, then there would be no sorrow.*

For prayer to be an effective form of meditation, it must be done in a quiet and conscious manner. All too often we are so caught up in our daily activities that we stop outside a temple or pray at home in a ritualistic manner without any concentration, while our mind is thinking of a million other things.

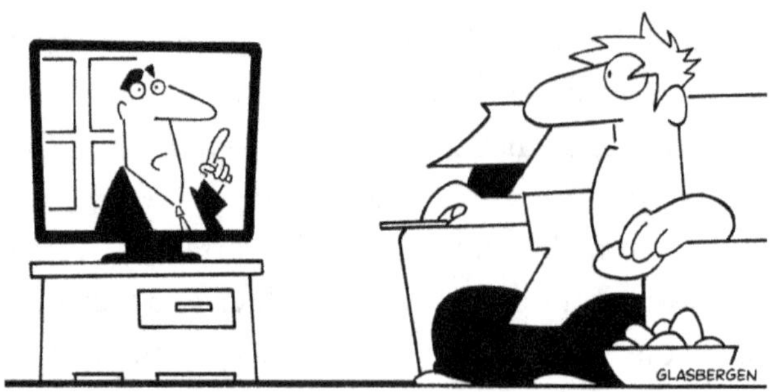

"For fast relief from stress, depression and anxiety,
four out of five doctors recommend money!"

Exercise as a stress buster

The next time you feel stressed, try this. Go out for an hour-long brisk walk or run, and see how you feel. It is almost impossible to feel stressed when you are in the midst of intense physical activity and the reason is simple. During a prolonged bout of continuous exercise, your brain releases chemicals called endorphins. These have morphine-like qualities, which act as painkillers and give the body a natural high. Now, why would anyone want to take illegal drugs when the best high is available free of cost, and is actually good for your health?

Several studies have shown that exercise is therapeutic for both depression and anxiety. In addition to its direct benefits in making you feel better, exercise has several other indirect benefits. A large number of patients tend to be relatively immobile after heart disease, due to anxiety. Once you start exercising, it's easier to get back to work, and often a big chunk of the patient's anxiety is lifted once they get back into the swing of things.

Depression

Mr Rajesh Chopra is a pleasant 65-year-old gentleman, who has a long-standing history of heart disease. Just like the Government of India has its five-year plans, he too seemed to have a five-year plan, but unfortunately for the wrong reason. After his first angioplasty in 1996, he had a repeat procedure in 2001, and again in 2006. He complained of chest pain again five years later in 2011. This time, after his angiography, it was decided to do a bypass surgery.

Initially, his progress was slow, but after a few months of intensive lifestyle changes he started feeling better. However, I noticed an inconsistent pattern in his recovery. There were days when he felt full of life and had no complaints, and there were days when even the slightest physical activity seemed to cause discomfort. Often his words were, '*Achha nahin lagta hai*'—I do not feel good. He also complained that he found it difficult to take in a 'full breath'. When I asked him to elaborate, he gave me a demonstration of taking in a deep breath and letting it out with an audible sigh. He was convinced that something was wrong with his lungs or his breathing. This is a situation I have come across many times in my practice, and after examining his chest I assured him that nothing was wrong. Frequent deep sighing is usually a sign of stress and/or anxiety, and is commonly seen in people who have undergone heart surgery. The challenging part is that if you tell the patient it's stress-related, he will typically get even more stressed about it, and the frequency will increase. Mr Chopra's symptoms did not correlate with his disease, and I suspected that there was something else causing him this discomfort. After detailed questioning, I realized that he was suffering from depression. Whenever he felt down, his cardiac symptoms acted up, and when he felt well, he was on top of the world.

In a vicious cycle, depression has been linked to heart disease. Studies have shown that depression can act as a causative factor for heart disease, and at the same time, a major cardiac event can cause depression. In fact, the risk for major depression can be as high as 40 per cent after a cardiac event. This depression can then lead to further development of heart disease, which is why I have labelled it as a vicious cycle.

Unfortunately, in our society, the word 'psychiatrist' has a stigma attached to it. The moment you suggest they seek professional help, most patients will tell you that their problem is not really that serious and they can take care of it themselves.

There is a commonly used standardized questionnaire to identify those with depression. It's called PHQ-9, which stands for patient health questionnaire. Take a moment and fill it out below. If you have scored more than 9 then you ought to be consulting with a mental health specialist. Depression need not be a permanent problem. Often, it's a phase that you may be going through, but getting the right help quickly can prevent it from becoming a long-term issue.

Patient Health Questionnaire-9 (PHQ 9)

OVER THE LAST 2 WEEKS, HOW OFTEN HAVE YOU BEEN BOTHERED BY ANY OF THE FOLLOWING PROBLEMS?	NOT AT ALL	SEVERAL DAYS	MORE THAN HALF THE DAYS	NEARLY EVERY DAY
1. Little interest or pleasure in doing things	0	1	2	3
2. Feeling down, depressed, or hopeless	0	1	2	3
3. Trouble falling or staying asleep, or sleeping too much	0	1	2	3
4. Feeling tired or having little energy	0	1	2	3
5. Poor appetite or overeating	0	1	2	3
6. Feeling bad about yourself – or that you are a failure or have let yourself or your family down	0	1	2	3
7. Trouble concentrating on things, such as reading the newspaper or watching television	0	1	2	3
8. Moving or speaking so slowly that other people may have noticed. Or the opposite – being so fidgety or restless that you have been moving around much more than usual	0	1	2	3
9. Thoughts that you would be better off dead, or of hurting yourself in some way	0	1	2	3
			Total score:	___

Interpretation of total score

Score	Interpretation
0-4	No depression
5-9	Mild depression
10-14	Moderate depression
15-19	Moderately severe depression
20-27	Severe depression

Yoga and heart disease

One of the most common questions I get asked is the role of yoga in the prevention and treatment of heart disease. Yoga is a vast and ancient tradition and science which teaches us to live life in a holistic manner. Since it is so vast it has come to mean different things to different people. For many it just means doing some stretches, while for others it means deep breathing a few times a day, and there are others who live their daily lives guided by the principles of yoga. In my opinion, a 'yogic' lifestyle will certainly lead to the prevention and control of heart disease. On the other hand, doing a few simple stretches and labelling them as yoga is often used as an excuse by most people to avoid physical activity and exercise.

Yoga has been part of the culture of the Indian sub-continent for centuries. Excavations done in the Indus Valley Civilization site have depicted people in yogic postures, suggesting its popularity even then. The most famous work on yoga is Patanjali's *Yoga Sutras*, which were published in the second century BC. One of the pioneers of the scientific study and implementation of yoga has been the Yoga Institute, in Santacruz in Mumbai. It's one of the oldest in the country, founded by Shri Yogendraji, in 1918. In 2004, the Yoga Institute conducted and published a study titled *The Beneficial Effects of Yoga Lifestyle on Reversibility of Ischemic Heart Disease*. In this study they took 71 patients with heart disease and put them through a program based on the principles of yoga, including asanas, nutrition, exercise and stress management, for a period of one year. In other words, the emphasis was on a yogic lifestyle, and not just physical asanas. At the end of the year, they showed that these patients had significantly improved their cardiac parameters and many had shown 'reversal' of their heart disease.

Gulistan Carpenter (popularly known as Gul maa by her students) has been teaching yoga to heart patients for over a decade, and has worked wonders with them. Most of the information I share with you now I have learned through Gulistan, and the institute.

The yogic way of life is based on four principles

- *Aahar or diet:* A balanced vegetarian diet. The emphasis though, is not just on the food content; it also needs to be prepared and eaten in a quiet and happy state of mind.
- *Vihar or recreation:* It's important to cultivate a hobby different from your profession. In addition, a daily brisk walk takes the mind of your routine chores and is recommended.
- *Aachar or behaviour:* We need to learn to 'respond' to life situations rather than 'react'. Our daily routine needs to be one of discipline and consistency.
- *Vichaar or thoughts:* Divine and positive thoughts will help shape our attitude and approach to life.

Three-step approach

I asked Gulistan what she felt were the most important aspects of yoga, which could be easily followed on a daily basis to prevent and reverse heart disease (apart from diet and physical activity). According to her, meditation, relaxation, and pranayama would be the three practices which could be done daily and lead to great results.

a) Meditation

Meditation has been described earlier, and I would like to emphasize that daily practise has shown to give excellent results in our patients, especially in the reduction of stress. Gulistan feels that it is very difficult for most people to remain thought-free (not thoughtless—that, people find easy!) during the meditation session, so it may be easier to channelize the thoughts in a positive direction. She suggested two different methods by which we can do this: while meditating, focus on the breath at the tip of your nostrils. Follow the breath as it passes through your nostrils, throat, and enters your lungs. Just focus on the breath. Do not in any way alter your breathing pattern. No forced breathing or deep breathing.

Another method is to think peaceful thoughts, or to recite a short mantra of your choosing. It could be as simple as, 'I am a pure soul, I am a peaceful soul.' After all, the word yoga itself means the union of an individual soul to the supreme soul.

b) Relaxation—shavasana

Our patients finish each yoga session with shavasana, which literally means corpse pose. I see them lying on the mat, with their arms and legs slightly apart, a beatific expression on their face. Remember, shavasana isn't a way to go to sleep. Rather, it's a progressive muscular relaxation, which helps you achieve a feeling of 'letting go'. It's a state of relaxed wakefulness that has many physiological benefits. Your heart rate and blood pressure are lowered, as is your rate of breathing. Follow these simple steps to do shavasana:

1. Find a nice quiet place and lie down on your back, with your feet apart and your hands slightly away from your body.
2. Consciously 'let go' and imagine that you are sinking into the floor. Keep your face totally relaxed, teeth unclenched, and eyes shut.
3. Give yourself conscious instructions to relax each body part one at a time. Start with your feet, calf muscles, thighs, shoulders, arms, and fingers. Feel your body going totally limp and light.
4. Visualize your heart and the blood flowing smoothly in your arteries without any blockages.
5. After the body is in shavasana for about 10–15 minutes, slowly bring some 'life' back by wriggling your toes and fingers. Turn on your side and gradually sit up and open your eyes.

c) Pranayama

This is a Sanskrit word which means 'extension of life force'. There are several different techniques of pranayama, and I will describe one of the easier ones which you can incorporate in your daily life.

Anulom vilom

This is a Sanskrit phrase which means alternate nostril breathing. According to Gulistan, this is considered to be the 'king of pranayamas'. It is supposed to purify the energy channels in our body, known as *nadis*. It has physical, mental, emotional and spiritual health benefits. Follow these simple steps to perform Anulom vilom:

- Sit on a chair with your feet shoulder-width apart and firmly planted on the floor. You can also sit in a cross-legged position on the ground if you prefer.
- With your right thumb, close your right nostril. With your right nostril shut, breathe in from your left nostril.
- Once you breathe in, close your left nostril with your index and middle fingers. After you have closed your left nostril, remove your thumb from the right nostril, and breathe out through it.
- Now inhale from the right nostril, and exhale from the left, and continue this sequence. Remember to close one nostril before you open the other. Please do not hold your breath.
- Keep your face totally relaxed, and do not exert any force. It is better to put a cushion or a pillow to support your back while doing this. Start with two minutes, and gradually build up to five, without getting breathless or fatigued.

In summary, a yogic lifestyle is not merely performing a few asanas, but living all aspects of your life with a higher level of consciousness. Dr Jayadeva Yogendra, the Director of the Yoga Institute (and son of the founder), had this to say about how to lead our lives: 'The enemy of cardiac patients is not just diabetes, cholesterol and blood pressure, but it is also crass materialism, selfishness, egotism, and negative emotions. We will have to turn our steps in the direction of a spiritual life if we want to live long, healthy, and happy lives.'

Faith and healing

One of my most vivid memories dates back to January 24, 2001. It was the day of Mauni Amavasya (night of no-moon), during the Kumbh Mela in Allahabad. The Kumbh Mela is the largest gathering of humanity anywhere in the world, and takes place in Allahabad once every 12 years. The 2001 mela was a Maha Kumbh, which takes place once in 144 years, and thus even more special. A twist of fate had placed me in the middle of the mela, and at 3 a.m. on a moonless night I began the long walk from the campground to the Ganges for a holy dip. Most people were fascinated by the warrior tribes of Naga Sadhus (naked holy men), but my attention was caught by the hundreds of frail old men and women who were walking in this sea of humanity. Many of them looked like they could barely walk a few feet, and yet they possessed this extraordinary faith which allowed them to walk for hours in near darkness on unstable pontoon bridges. They were able to do this purely on the strength of their faith and belief.

I mention this story here because time and again I have seen how faith and belief can cure a patient. Stressors, both small and big, are present in most peoples' lives, but it's their perception of these stressors which alter their responses. Their ability to deal with them is greatly influenced by their own belief system. If they want to get better, then all the mental stress can be dealt with; and conversely, if they don't want to get better, then there is no amount of medication or miracles that can help them. I have often heard surgeons comment that the patients who did not make it after surgery were not necessarily the ones whose disease was the most complex. The ones that did not make it were the ones who went into surgery 'believing' that they would never get better. One of my favourite lines is, 'You live your life in your mind.' A very large part of your ability to deal with disease is dependent on your thought process, and the only person who can control that is YOU.

Take-home messages

- Psychosocial factors, which include stress, depression, anxiety, anger, hostility, and social isolation have tremendous impact on heart disease risk.

- Stress is an integral part of daily life and cannot be totally avoided. However, our reaction to stress is more important and that is in our control.

- Meditation and exercise are great stress-management techniques.

- A yogic way of life, which includes the right Aahar, Vihar, Aachar, and Vichaar prevents stress and heart disease.

- Add a simple daily yoga practice to your routine, which includes meditation, relaxation, and pranayama.

15

Medication

(A bitter pill to swallow)

ONE AFTERNOON, WHILE I WAS PRACTICING IN THE US, ONE OF MY favourite patients, Sammy Giles, walked in and greeted me warmly. Sammy was a typical Southern gentleman, full of good manners and always very cheerful. After going through his latest reports, I asked him for a list of his current medications. He rattled off half the pharmacy, before suddenly stopping. Then he said, 'Doc, there is one more med, but for the life of me I can't remember the name.' Later that day, I got a call from Sammy, who very excitedly told me that the name of the medicine he had forgotten was the one he took for his memory. I laughed, and asked him to take a double dose for the day. While this sounds like a joke, it's a true story, and though it happened 15 years ago, I am glad I have not forgotten it!

While I may be guilty of cultural stereotyping, in my experience American patients are quite happy to pop a pill for everything (including memory), while Indian patients are on the other end of the scale, and want to do everything to avoid taking medicine. I often get asked whether it really is necessary to take a prescribed medicine, with much emphasis on the word 'really'. For most chronic conditions, such as blood pressure and cholesterol, I have a fairly standard answer: you need to achieve control of the parameters. If it can be done without pills, then that's fantastic, but it does not make sense to avoid the pill, and not have the values under control.

Pills for your heart

Medications prescribed for heart disease can be divided into two broad categories.

1. Medication that is taken to provide relief of symptoms and make you feel better.
2. Medication that helps reduce your risk of heart attack and death.

There are also drugs which do both of the above actions, and in general this kind of classification is applicable for all medical conditions. Let's take the example of paracetamol, sold under the trade name of Crocin. It's commonly taken to relieve a headache or fever, or as a mild painkiller. The moment you feel better, you stop taking it. It does not have long-term preventive effects on your body. On the other hand, heart patients are prescribed aspirin, not to make them 'feel' better, but as a blood thinner to prevent future chances of heart attack and death. Therefore, such a pill has to be taken on a daily basis, irrespective of how you currently feel. This is the reason why some heart patients are on lifelong drugs, even though their parameters are under control.

Generic versus trade names

One of the most confusing aspects of taking medications, both for patients and doctors, is the vast variety of drugs available and the number of companies that make each of them. Every drug has a scientific name, also known as the generic name. In countries with strict patent laws, for the first several years of its life, each drug is manufactured only by the company which discovers and patents it, before it goes 'off-patent'. For example, in the last 15 years or so, the bestselling statin, atorvastatin, was made only by Pfizer and was known as Lipitor. On the other hand, in India, there are at least 30 versions of atorvastatin, with different names. Multiply that by the number of different cardiac drugs in the marketplace, and you literally need a computer program (there are several available today) to keep track of all the available permutations and combinations. Aamir Khan, on his show *Satyamev Jayate,* discussed the topic of generic drugs and how doctors are guilty of prescribing expensive ones when cheaper versions are available. While there is some truth in that, one also needs to be aware of the reputation of the company manufacturing the drug. Like in all other consumables, it is easy to save money by cutting corners, but this can be particularly dangerous in the area of medications. I advise my patients to select the cheapest version of the drug as long as it's made by a reputed company.

Over the next few pages, I would like to talk about the most common cardiac medications that almost every person with heart disease will be or should be taking. Of course, there are several more, but let's focus on the most important ones for the moment. It's easy to remember them as A, B, C.

- A for aspirin
- B for blood pressure meds
- C for cholesterol meds

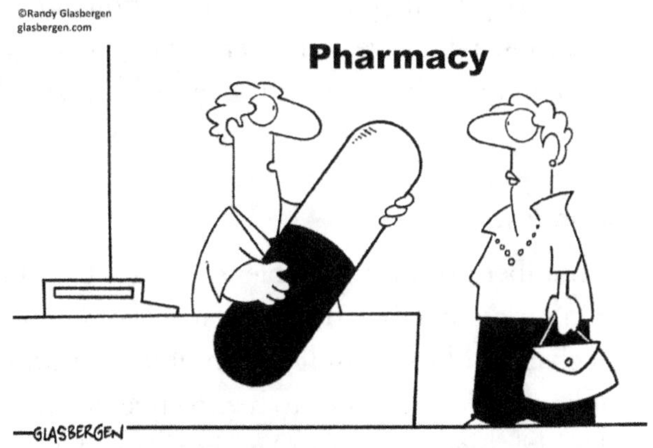

"Each capsule contains your medication, plus a treatment for each of its side effects."

Aspirin

Aspirin is actually the trade name of the drug technically known as acetyl salicylic acid. It was called aspirin by the German drug manufacturer Bayer, and has become so well known that, for most users, aspirin has actually become the generic name, much like Xerox. Of all the cardiac drugs, this is the most important, with maximum research done on its effectiveness.

Aspirin acts by preventing the tiny blood cells called platelets from sticking together and forming a thrombus, and therefore is colloquially known as a blood thinner. This prevents heart attacks, and that's why aspirin is considered among the best cardiac drugs to reduce mortality. All patients with a diagnosis of heart disease are recommended to take aspirin lifelong, though the dosage varies from 325 mg a day, to 75 mg a day, also known as a baby aspirin.

The side effects of aspirin are ironically related to its good effects. Due to its blood-thinning properties, it can lead to bleeding in areas such as the digestive system, causing or aggravating stomach ulcers, or bleeding from the rectum. Luckily these are not very common and most people tolerate it very well. One of the relatively common side effects is acidity, which is why doctors recommend taking it after a meal. To decrease acidity many manufacturers coat the aspirin, which makes it dissolve slower in the stomach and decreases acidity. The most common aspirin in the Indian market is Ecosprin.

In addition to aspirin, there are two other blood thinners that are commonly used: clopidogrel and prasugrel. Their actions are very similar to that of aspirin, and those who have had a stent or bypass surgery should be taking both, aspirin and clopidogrel (or prasugrel) for a period of one year at least.

Blood pressure medication

There are a large number of drugs available to control blood pressure, and they can be given in various combinations. The most common drugs are beta blockers, calcium channel blockers and ACE inhibitors. They have different mechanisms of action, and have shown to be effective in a variety of cardiac conditions besides high blood pressure. Another class of drugs that is very popular is diuretics, more commonly called 'water pills', since they help remove excess fluid from the body. They help to control blood pressure and are also used in heart failure.

Most people with high blood pressure are afraid to start medication, since they have this belief that once you start on BP pills, you need to take them for life. Actually, this is not true. What is true is that you need to keep your BP under control if you want to avoid a heart attack and stroke, and as explained at the start of this chapter, it would be wonderful to have it under control 'naturally', but if that cannot be done, then medication is necessary. Let me illustrate this with a case study.

Anand Sinha is a 55-year-old corporate head honcho who led a very sedentary lifestyle. His only physical activity was walking from the entrance of his building to get into his chauffeur-driven car, and from the elevator to his corner office, which had a view of the sea. Since he was on the top of the corporate ladder, clients came to his office for meetings, rather than him needing to go anywhere. Time is money (or so he believed), therefore he ate his lunch, and on busy days, his dinner too, at his desk. He did get some physical activity at night: while watching TV, he had to get up and make trips to the kitchen for snacks since the house-help was asleep. When he came for his annual check-up, he was 18 kg overweight, had a BP of 170/100, and had high cholesterol levels. I made him relax and checked it again, but it was the same. I usually do not like to begin medication before a reasonable trial of lifestyle changes, but at these levels his BP was dangerous and he was at risk for a stroke. I started him on a moderate dose of amlodipine (a calcium channel blocker) and ramipril(an ACE inhibitor), and asked him to see me after two weeks. I also discussed a detailed lifestyle modification plan, and told him that it was the only way he had a hope of getting off the medications.

When I met him after two weeks, his BP was 150/90, which is still high, but better than before. Over time though, he began losing weight and his BP numbers came within control. As he continued losing weight, we were able to knock off one of the medications. After a year he had lost nearly 15 kg, and was walking daily to work (with his car tailing him, much to the amusement of his driver). He was now able to control his BP without any medication.

As you saw in this case, it is possible to get off drugs once you start them, as long as you get the numbers right. A lot also matters on your starting point. In other words, those who are worse off to start with (from a lifestyle point of view) have a much greater room for improvement.

Statins

These are a family of cholesterol-lowering drugs which contain an all-star cast comprising simvastatin, atorvastatin, and rozuvastatin. The reason I call it an all-star cast is that these have been the largest-selling drugs in the world over the past two decades. Just as penicillin was a wonder drug in the 1940s and aspirin in the early 1900s, in the mid 1990s statins achieved this status, and have maintained it since.

Their primary effect is to lower total cholesterol and LDL cholesterol. Depending on the type of statin and the strength of the drug, it can do so in very large numbers. Statins act by blocking off one of the enzymes required in the production of cholesterol. In other words, they slow down the cholesterol-making factory in the liver. They act quickly, and by the same token, they lose their effects quickly. Often patients start taking statins and when they test their lipid profile again, they will find a significant drop. They then assume that all is well, and stop taking the medicine, only to find out during their next test that they are back to square one.

The early statin trials had thousands of patients in them, and researchers found a reduction in the number of deaths and heart attacks in those on statins. However, this reduction did not correlate completely with the lipid-lowering effects of the statins—in other words, the decrease in heart attacks seemed disproportionate to the fall in the LDL cholesterol levels. Scientists have put this down to the pleiotropic effects of statins. Pleiotropic effects of a drug refer to actions of the medicine other than those it was developed for. It is theorized that statins lead to stabilization of the atherosclerotic plaque and thereby reduce heart attacks, apart from their LDL-lowering abilities. Remember, heart attacks occur when plaques rupture, so anything which helps stabilize the plaque will reduce the number of attacks. This is the reason why all heart patients are recommended statins lifelong, even if their cholesterol levels are naturally low. Speaking of pleiotropic effects, did you know that Viagra was actually developed as a blood pressure drug, before an interesting side effect was noted?

Any drug which is a blockbuster will have its fair share of detractors and I think statins are the drugs which people love to hate the most. All over the internet, you will see articles plastered on how bad they are and how they should be stopped immediately. My personal approach to the statin controversy (and all the others which keep popping up in the medical world) is to evaluate all the evidence at hand and then take a call. When reviewing any drug, it is vital to look at the benefit-to-risk ratio of the drug—that is, what are the benefits and do they outweigh any potential risks. Looked at in that manner, statins are overwhelmingly effective drugs, and until there is any new evidence suggesting otherwise, I would recommend you take them.

The most common side effects of statins are related to the muscles and liver. Some patients complain of generalized muscle weakness or cramping when on statins. One of the tests to check if the muscle weakness is due to statins is a blood test to measure creatine kinase. This is a muscle enzyme which may be elevated due to statins, but bear in mind that the recommendations say that you should consider stopping the statin only if this enzyme is more than 10 times its normal limit. The other enzymes which are sometimes elevated with statin use are the liver enzymes SGOT and SGPT. If their levels are more than three times normal, it may be an indication to stop the drug.

Natural statins

Red yeast rice is rice that has been fermented by red yeast. It has been used in China since centuries, and recently it has been converted to capsule form and sold as a natural supplement. Red yeast rice has shown to have cholesterol-lowering properties similar to statins, and in preliminary reports seems to be quite safe. It might be an alternative for those with high cholesterol (and do not have heart disease), who do not want to take a statin. However, since it's sold as a supplement, its manufacturing is not as tightly monitored as those of statins. Therefore, if you do take it, make sure it's from a reputed company with strict quality control.

What about the side effects of cardiac drugs?

The other day, one of my patients complained to me that pharma companies were making the tablets too brittle. I asked him how he had come to that conclusion, and he told me that he was having a hard time snipping off the edges of the pills with his scissor. Naturally I had to ask him why he was doing something that bizarre, and he replied with a big grin, 'Doc, I want to cut off the side effects of the drug.' Okay, that did not really happen. Actually, it was a joke that one of my friends who works as an intensivist (ICU doctor) sent me. (But the story about the memory pill at the start of the chapter is true!)

In all seriousness, patients have every right to be concerned about the side effects of medications since they certainly do exist. It would be best to classify these into two categories: common, but not life-threatening side effects, and those which are life-threatening, but not common. If they are common and life-threatening, then the drug would be banned, so you need not worry about those.

Doctors often face a dilemma when discussing side effects, or adverse effects, with patients. On the one hand, it is their duty to inform the patient about anything that might affect his or her body, but on the other, there is a tendency for some patients to 'feel' the side effects the moment they are told about it. If you go through the information in any drug packaging and read through every possible side effect, then I doubt you would take a single pill. The reason they mention even the rarest possibility is to make sure the pharma companies are legally covered.

In my opinion, a balance is needed, and I believe in discussing common side effects, as well as dangerous side effects, if there are any. For example, ACE inhibitors (common generic names are ramipril, lisinopril, and captopril) tend to give some patients a dry cough. While this is not dangerous, it can certainly be irritating. If it's reasonably bearable then I would advise you to continue with the medication since it usually gets better with time. If not, there are other drugs which can be taken instead. On the other hand, if you see fresh blood in your stools or urine, it could be due to the effects of blood thinners, which may need to be stopped at once. Excessive blood thinning may lead to bleeding, which can be particularly dangerous if it happens to an artery in the brain. Luckily, most of the drugs in the cardiac armamentarium are relatively safe and rarely do we see any serious side effects.

I met Mrs Geeta Saraiya during a consultation for her high cholesterol. She was 46 years old and had LDL cholesterol of 201, which is very high. I spoke to her about various lifestyle changes that she needed to make, and also advised her to start medication. She seemed very hesitant to do so, and when I asked her why, she told me that if she started medication at this young age, she would need to take it long term. Her concern was that when taken long term, the medication would 'lose its effect'. This is a concern I have heard from many different patients and I would like to assure you that this does not happen. Taking a medicine long term does not make it lose its effect.

Commonly-used heart medications, their uses and side effects

MEDICATION USED	CLASS OF DRUG	COMMON GENERIC NAMES	COMMON TRADE NAMES	USED FOR	SIDE EFFECTS
Blood pressure	Beta blockers	Atenolol, Metoprolol, Carvedilol	Aten, Seloken, Betaloc, Cardivas	BP, angina, heart failure, after heart attack	Airways (breathing) spasm, fatigue, slow heart rate
	ACE inhibitors/ ARB	Ramipril, Losartan, Telmisartan, Valsartan	Cardace, Losar, Telma, Diovan	BP, heart failure, after heart attack	Dry cough, increase in potassium levels, rash
	Calcium channel blockers	Amlodipine, Diltiazem, Nifedipine	Amlopin, Dilzem, Depin, Calcigard	BP, angina	Ankle swelling, low BP
	Diuretics (water pills)	Frusomide, HCTZ, Indapamide	Lasix, Esidrex, Natrilix	BP, heart failure	Electrolyte imbalance, excess urination
Blood thinners		Aspirin, Clopidogrel, Prasugrel	Ecosprin, Plavix, Deplatt, Prax	Preventive measure for anyone with heart disease	Bleeding in stools, urine or gastrointestinal system
Anti-angina	Nitrates	Isosorbide dinitrate, isosorbide mononitrate	Sorbitrate, Imdur	Angina	Lightheadedness, low BP
Anti-cholesterol	Statins	Simvastatin, Atorvastatin, Rozuvastatin	Zosta, Aztor, Storvas, Rozuvas, Razel	Cholesterol-lowering and preventive measure for anyone with heart disease	Muscle aches and elevated liver enzymes

Medicines work only if you take them

Whenever I see patients in the hospital prior to discharge, I discuss their homecare plan with them. One of the areas I touch upon is medication, and my advice is simple. Please take your medication as prescribed, regularly and on time. Clearly, this is common sense, and I am not saying anything special, but it might shock you to know that 50 per cent of patients do not take their medications as prescribed over the long term. Which means that there are one out of two chances that you are one of them! I jokingly tell my patients that if you must reduce your medications, at least talk to me first. I can then stop your least important pill rather than you doing it on your own and risk stopping the most important one.

Another common occurrence in my experience is a mismatch between pills prescribed and the ones actually taken by the patient. This usually happens in cases of long-standing medical history and repeated visits to doctors, especially visits to multiple doctors. Patients often end up taking two pills from the same family of drugs with different trade names. To prevent this from happening, I always recommend that you actually carry the physical strips of medicine with you to the doctor, as well as the written prescription, especially when you are taking several different pills.

Take-home messages

- Some cardiac medications are prescribed to provide long-term protection, while others are prescribed for immediate symptom relief.

- Blood thinners (aspirin) and cholesterol-reducing drugs (statins) need to be taken long term for those with heart disease. They have protective effects against heart attack and death.

- It is a myth that once you start blood pressure medications they need to be taken for life. If you achieve good BP control through lifestyle modification, you may be able to get off medication.

- Many patients tend to stop taking their medication without talking to their doctor. This is a dangerous practice and should be avoided.

16

Cardiac Rehabilitation

(Being better than before)

NEVER MAKE THE MISTAKE OF SHAKING HANDS WITH GURUNATH Nadkarni. he is 85 years old and has a vice-like grip that makes you wonder where he gets his strength from. It was a very different story a few years ago, when he was fighting for his life and could barely lift his hand, let alone use it to hold anything. In August 2010, at the age of 82, he underwent bypass surgery, in spite of having an extremely weak heart with a pumping capacity of 15 per cent. A few days after his surgery, his chest had to be cut open again due to complications, and he was 're-explored'. He spent an extended time in the ICU on life support and made it through thanks to his enormous fighting spirit and the medical care he received.

The first time he entered the Cardiac Rehabilitation Centre at the Asian Heart Institute, he came on a wheelchair and needed the support of a couple of people in order to stand. I distinctly remember helping him take his first steps, which actually were very few due to extreme weakness. Prolonged bed rest takes a huge toll on the body overall, especially the cardiovascular system, and this was compounded by advanced age. Most people would have given up at this stage, but not Mr Nadkarni. In his own words, he is a proud GSB (Goud Saraswat Brahmin), and with his trademark beret and ramrod straight walk, reminds me of an older generation of Maharashtrians whom you routinely see taking a brisk walk around Shivaji Park in Mumbai. He progressed step by painful step, and within a few weeks of cardiac rehabilitation, was able to walk on his own. Over a three-year period, he has greatly increased his capacity, and today is able to exercise for a total of 50 minutes on the treadmill and stationary bicycle. Isn't that truly amazing for any 85-year-old, let alone one who has had open heart surgery and started with a heart-pumping capacity of 15 per cent? His most recent 2-D echo showed that this number has increased to 30 per cent, which is still lower than normal, but is double of where he started. Over the past 15 years I have come across hundreds of such inspirational cases who have benefited from cardiac rehabilitation.

What is cardiac rehabilitation?

The term cardiac rehabilitation, as defined by the World Health Organization (WHO), refers to coordinated, multifaceted interventions designed to optimize a cardiac patient's physical, psychological, and social functioning, in addition to stabilizing, slowing, or even reversing the progression of the underlying atherosclerotic processes, thereby reducing risk of further disease.

That's a complicated sounding statement, and in simple words, cardiac rehab is a comprehensive program which helps a patient recover from heart disease, and prevent recurrence of the disease. The main goals of the program are:

- To get a person back to normalcy as quickly and safely as possible after a heart attack, angioplasty or bypass surgery.
- To institute lifestyle changes and regular monitoring to reduce future risk of cardiac events.
- To improve the psychological well being of the cardiac patient.

Life begins after heart disease

Heart disease can be a life-changing event. Whether it's a positive or negative life-changer often depends on the attitude of the patient. Many patients never fully recover from the blow, and end up being 'cardiac cripples'. They go home from hospital and remain in bed all day long. Many of them are physically okay, but have a perception that since they have had a heart problem, they should get as much rest as possible. Prolonged rest reduces their physical capacity, and when they do try and get out of bed, they get tired easily.

This leads to a drop in confidence, which leads to further slowing down of activity, causing a deterioration in physical capability, which further reduces confidence, and the vicious cycle continues.

However, heart disease can be a positive life-changing event. If appropriate care is taken, most people not only recover, but also go on to improve their quality of life to a higher level than before. After any heart event, post-care and rehabilitation is a vital part of the treatment. A structured cardiac rehabilitation program is crucial to get the patient on the path to recovery, and to prevent further illness.

What does the research show?

Extensive research has revealed that, when compared with usual medical care, patients who undergo cardiac rehabilitation show a reduction of 20 per cent in total death and 26 per cent in cardiac deaths. In fact, such is its importance that leading cardiology associations like the American Heart Association have classified it as a Class I recommendation, on par with other life-saving measures, such as a daily aspirin dose. In other words, it's a therapy which must be recommended to all cardiac patients.

When does cardiac rehabilitation start?

The sooner the better. The program should start the moment the patient is discharged from hospital. After bypass surgery, we usually begin the process within 10-14 days, if there are no complications. Similarly, after an angioplasty, cardiac rehabilitation can be begun within a few days if there are no complications. In fact, for some patients who are clinically stable, it can even begin while they are in the hospital.

What happens during the program?

Often patients and their family members walk into a cardiac rehab centre and get the impression that they are in a gym. This is because they see several people exercising at the same time. Actually, exercise forms only one component of the program, but it's the most visible one. In reality, cardiac rehabilitation looks at every aspect of the patient's risk profile, and works at keeping it to a minimum.

Initially, the patient is thoroughly evaluated from a medical, physical and emotional standpoint. Following the evaluation, an individualized program of exercise, nutrition, and stress reduction is planned. The patient visits the centre thrice a week, and exercises using portable heart monitoring equipment known as telemetry. With the help of this special equipment, the ECG is continuously transmitted to the monitoring station wirelessly while the person is exercising. This ensures that the optimal amount of exercise is performed in the safest manner possible.

In addition to exercise, the patient's risk factors are charted out and goals are set for each of them. These are evaluated at regular intervals to ensure optimum risk factor management. Since the patient visits the program frequently, the team is able to fine-tune his or her medications to achieve perfect control over most cardiac parameters. Let's take the example of blood pressure. Typically, the patient visits his or her doctor once in four to six weeks, and medications are changed based on one reading taken in six weeks. This may or may not be truly representative of the patient's usual pressure. On the other hand, the patient visits the rehab centre thrice a week, and BP is charted several times at each visit. This allows 'titration' of medications to achieve aggressive risk factor control—not just ordinary control.

Besides exercise and risk factor reduction, diet and stress management form an integral component of the process. Again, the frequency of visits allows the dietician to tailor a meal plan which suits the patient's health and cultural needs and modifications can be made as needed. Stress management is done through a variety of methods, which often include yoga, meditation and group support.

Group support helps

They say, 'You don't know how it feels till you have walked in another person's shoes'. I am sure patients often think this when they are listening to advice from doctors. Dr Sharma (name changed) was a senior cardiac surgeon who had himself undergone bypass surgery in the past. One day while he was on ward rounds, one of the patients was complaining of pain after surgery. Dr Sharma did his best to explain that this pain was to be expected but was temporary. The patient wasn't too convinced and said, 'Doctor, that's easy for you to say, you haven't been operated.' Dr. Sharma then dramatically removed his lab coat, and opened up the front buttons of his shirt to reveal the long, vertical surgical scar on his chest, a telltale sign of bypass surgery. While the patient was staring dumbstruck, he smiled and said, 'I believe I have earned the right to be giving you real life advice.' After that, the patient stopped complaining about pain.

Heart disease can be very traumatic. Some patients go through a short period of depression when they first get out of the hospital, wondering if they will ever be 'normal' again, and be able to resume their usual activities. The support of family and doctors is extremely important, but often the best guidance comes from other patients who have gone through the same experience. In the cardiac rehabilitation program, patients share experiences with others who have had the same problems. This group support goes a long way in providing reassurance to the patient and is an integral part of the program.

Mental confidence gets a boost

Ashok Gowariker is a towering individual. He is 6 feet 4 inches tall, and though he is 78 years old, he barely looks a day beyond 60. He was in the police force in the early part of his life, and regular physical activity had kept him fit. In his later years, he entered the film industry and teamed up with his son Ashutosh to produce blockbuster hits, including *Lagaan*, *Swades*, and *Jodha Akbar*. He used to walk daily, and on one of his walks, he noticed a pull on the right side of his chest, near the shoulder. That started a series of investigations, which ultimately led to a bypass surgery in June 2013. After surgery, Mr Gowariker started in cardiac rehab, but was tentative at first. Gradually, we were able to progress him, and as his physical condition improved, so did his state of mind. Once, during a consultation, he confided in me that the greatest benefit he got from cardiac rehab was mental confidence. He is now back to 'action, lights, cameras', and we look forward to many more hits from his production house. In my opinion, mental confidence is one of the greatest benefits of good cardiac rehabilitation, and helps a person to get back to a 'better than before' state. When patients are able to greatly improve their physical capacity, it also translates into them feeling more confident about their future.

Who can benefit from cardiac rehabilitation?

Quite frankly, anyone who has suffered from heart disease, or is at risk for heart disease, can benefit from a structured cardiac rehabilitation program. This includes those who have undergone:

- Heart attack
- Bypass surgery
- Angioplasty
- Angiography showing blockages
- Heart failure
- Heart valve replacement
- Angina

Cure the disease, don't just repair it

After a surgery or plasty, many patients ask me if they 'have' to undergo cardiac rehab. My answer to them is simple: surgery or angioplasty is a repair job to take care of the blockage and get you out of immediate danger. The cardiac rehab process is a cure for the problem. It gets to the root of why you had heart disease in the first place, and works out solutions to reduce future risk.

Over the past 17 years, I have come across more than 10,000 patients who have benefited from cardiac rehab, and would strongly recommend that every person with heart disease go through a good rehab program.

Take-home messages

- ℗ The goals of cardiac rehabilitation are to get a person back to normal as quickly and safely as possible after a cardiac event, and to reduce future risk of heart disease.

- ℗ The program consists of comprehensive cardiac risk reduction, along with lifestyle modification.

- ℗ It is an integral part of care after a heart attack, bypass surgery, or angioplasty, and must be done.

- ℗ Cardiac rehabilitation instils a great deal of physical and mental confidence in the patient.

17

Women and Heart Disease

(Women are not from Venus)

SABINA GUPTA, BY ALL DEFINITIONS, WAS THE PROTOTYPE OF THE SUCCESSFUL modern woman. At the age of 53, she ran a thriving confectionary business while taking care of her family at the same time. Sabina's business supplied cakes and other bakery items to more than 300 clients daily, and she led a very active work life. In between raising a family and taking care of business, she also found time to get in a daily hour of exercise. Her exercise routine varied, but included tennis, running and Iyengar yoga. Of late she had begun noticing a slight amount of breathlessness on climbing stairs, and felt as if 'something was pulling her back'. She had a very strong family history of heart

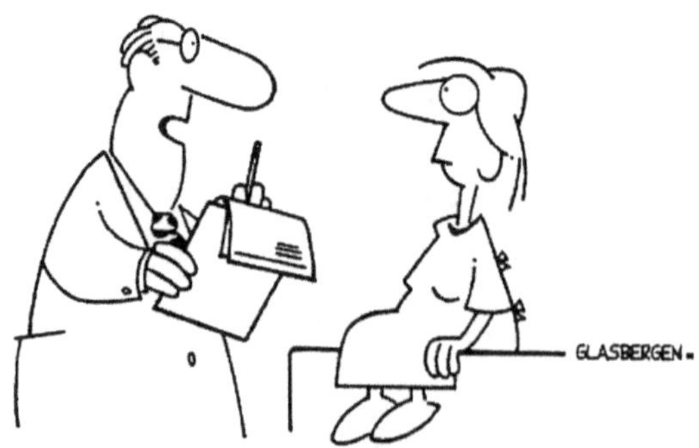

**"Many women fear the word 'menopause'
so I prefer to call it Puberty Part II."**

disease, with several members on both her parents' side suffering at an early age. Even then, heart disease was the last thing on her mind, since she figured she was a woman, and in any case, she did not have any chest discomfort.

The chest discomfort did happen. One evening she was having a party on her building terrace, and like all good hostesses was quite stressed about it, wanting everything to be perfect. At first she felt a pain on the right side of her chest, which then spread to her neck. Luckily there was a doctor at the party who recommended that she be taken to the hospital immediately and get tested for a heart attack. The enzyme test (for a heart attack) was negative, and after a few days of rest, she underwent a dobutamine stress echo test. This is an advanced stress test in which the heart rate is raised via a medication given intravenously in place of exercise. Women often tend to have false readings on regular stress tests, and are recommended a dobutamine stress echo or stress thallium instead. Her test was positive, and the next step was an angiography. Sabina Gupta, who thought women do not get heart disease, had eight blockages show up on her angiography, and needed a bypass surgery.

Whenever I address a group of women on health issues, the first question I ask them is what they think is the number one cause of death in women. Most of them are usually very shy and do not reply, but those who do invariably say breast cancer. Actually, heart disease is the leading cause of death in women worldwide, and in India too. This is the reason I decided to dedicate a separate chapter on women and heart disease, to highlight its importance. I was surprised to see the statistics which showed that heart disease (to be more accurate, cardiovascular disease, which includes stroke) is the leading cause of death in India, across all categories of men and women: rural, urban, economically advanced states and economically backward states. Clearly, it's not just a disease of the rich. What is shocking though, and a severe indictment of our healthcare system, is that diarrhoea is the second leading cause of death in women in India. Yes, you read that right. And just in case you doubt that (as much as I did when I first read it), let me inform you that it's from the official Government of India report, and here is the citation: *Registrar General of India and Million Death Study Investigators: Final Report on Causes of Death in India 2001-2003. New Delhi; 2009.*

Getting back to cardiovascular disease—not only is it the leading cause of death in India for women, but it also kills roughly three times more women than all cancers put together. So why is it that we see such few women in the cardiac wing of hospitals as compared to men?

Where are all the women?

Even though the number of women with heart disease is similar to men, you will find very few women in the cardiac wards of hospitals. There are several reasons for this, both medical and social. From the medical standpoint, heart disease has traditionally never been thought to be a woman's disease, so when a woman does complain of symptoms such as breathlessness, everyone around her, including doctors, will not think of heart disease as a first diagnosis. The pattern of symptoms exhibited by women is also slightly different from men, which also tends to delay the diagnosis. The other reasons why women receive less treatment are unfortunately social. Indian women are probably the hardest working and most selfless human beings in the world. They play the role of homemaker, wage-earner, mother, wife, daughter, and daughter-in-law all at the same time. They take care of everybody around them, except themselves. Their health is the most neglected, and unfortunately this starts from childhood. Imagine a situation in a household where a 55-year-old man and his 50-year-old wife are both diagnosed with triple vessel disease and are in need of bypass surgery, costing close to 4 lakh rupees. No prizes for guessing which member of the family will get the surgery if there are limited funds. Quite frankly, in many cases, even when the funds are not limited the story is the same.

Women are different from men

The symptoms of heart disease that women experience are often different from those that men feel. Typically, women do not get the classic pattern of angina with pain in the left side of the chest. They are more likely to have atypical angina, in which they could experience discomfort in the shoulders, back, and neck. Also, shortness of breath is often the first and only presenting symptom, making diagnosis tricky, since there are several causes of shortness of breath. When women present with these symptoms to the doctor, and they settle down quickly, they are often dismissed as non-cardiac and further investigations are not carried out.

The risk factors for heart disease are the same among men and women, but they do differ slightly in terms of importance. Diabetes is even more dangerous in women than in men, and women with diabetes are three to five times more likely to have heart disease than those without diabetes. In younger women, smoking tends to be an extremely dangerous risk factor, and all patients should be questioned about tobacco use. In most parts of India, it's considered a social taboo for women to smoke, and because of this, doctors often hesitate to broach the subject. After asking several women patients whether they smoke and getting reactions ranging from amusement to downright dirty looks, I have learned a new trick. I do ask the question, but ask it in the negative: 'You don't take tobacco in any form, do you?' I have found that this works much better, especially among older ladies who tend to get offended if you ask them about tobacco or smoking. Having said that, you will be surprised to know that 20 per cent of all adult Indian women consume tobacco in some form. Most of this is the smokeless variety, but cigarette consumption among urban women is definitely on the rise.

Women tend to have a higher level of good cholesterol (HDL) than men, but this tends to drop after menopause. Speaking of menopause, up to a decade ago, menopausal women routinely received hormone replacement therapy (HRT). When I was working in the US, we used to prescribe HRT to all post-menopausal women as a heart disease prevention strategy, irrespective of their risk profile. Unfortunately, studies over the last decade have shown that not only is this not beneficial, it may also actually be harmful.

Emotional support

Harshad Desai is a rare breed. I was struck by the care he takes of his wife each time I saw him sitting among all the women in the waiting lounge of the Cardiac Rehabilitation Centre. His wife, Jyotsna Desai, had bypass surgery in July 2005, and subsequently enrolled in cardiac rehabilitation as part of her routine care. Mr Desai would accompany her for all her visits to the hospital, even when she was capable of travelling on her own. I found her recovery to be much faster than most of our other female patients. In all my years of working in India and the US, I have noticed that when a man is the patient, his spouse always accompanies him to the doctor, usually with other family members in attendance. However, when the woman is the patient, the reverse is usually not true, and she often shows up for follow-up treatment alone or with a maid. The happy ending to the Desai story is that after dutifully accompanying his wife for over two years, Mr Desai himself joined our preventive program, and is in much better health. A happy family is one that takes care of each other's heart.

Women are so used to playing the role of caregiver that they almost feel guilty when it comes to taking care of themselves. This is also one of the reasons why they often receive less than adequate treatment even after being diagnosed with heart disease. Research has shown that depression is a more potent risk factor for heart disease in women than in men. It contributes directly to plaque formation and indirectly as well, since those who are depressed do not follow their treatment guidelines well. So, for all the men reading this book, I hope you have not skipped this chapter, and from now on pay more attention to the health of the women around you. And ladies, do remember to take care of your hearts—they are very precious.

Take-home messages

- Heart disease is the leading cause of death in women all over the world, and in India too.

- Unfortunately, the diagnosis of heart disease is often missed out in women, which is why they get less care than men.

- Women usually don't get the typical symptoms of angina. Shortness of breath is often the only symptom they get.

18

Sex and Heart Disease

(Getting back to intimacy)

I REGULARLY CONDUCT LECTURES FOR PATIENTS AND THEIR RELATIVES, during which time various aspects of heart disease are discussed, followed by a Q and A session. I was conducting one of these, and when it was time for questions, one of the younger patients in the room shot his hand up. His question was, 'Doctor, when can I start having sex?' There was pin-drop silence in the room, and I could see that his wife sitting next to him was visibly embarrassed. Most of the people in the room were between the age of 50 and 75, and they were clearly uncomfortable too. I did answer the question, and at the end of the session, the patient walked up to me and asked if he had said something wrong. When I thought about it, I realized that this is a topic which we should be addressing with each and every patient, but a false sense of coyness comes over us, and we pretend the issue does not exist.

Sexual activity after heart disease

After suffering from a heart attack or undergoing a bypass surgery or angioplasty, most patients are very apprehensive about resuming their sex life. Since sex tends to be a taboo topic, most of them do not even discuss it with their spouse, let alone their doctor, and consequently a fear develops around the subject. The fear is centred on the effects of sexual activity and of 'straining the heart'. This fear is exacerbated by movies, which often depict a person having a heart attack while in the middle of sexual activity.

Some famous people who actually died during sexual activity perpetuate the myth. Nelson Rockefeller, the Vice-President of the United States, died in 1979 while in the 'intimate company' of a young female aide. In reality, the amount of effort required for sexual activity is similar to that required to climb two flights of stairs, or walking at a pace of 4–5 km/hour. This may disappoint many men who might have overestimated their sexual prowess. Studies conducted (primarily in young married men), have shown that the heart rate rarely exceeds 130 beats/minute during sexual activity, and the physiological workload on the body is in the range of 3–5 METS. The term METS refers to the oxygen consumption of the body, with 1 MET representing the consumption at rest. In other words, during sexual activity, oxygen consumption is three to five times that of rest. While this is a small workload for the hearts of most young or middle-aged people, it can represent a higher workload for older individuals, and they need to be counselled accordingly. It's a failing on most doctors' parts that we do not discuss this subject, especially with our older patients. For some reason, we just assume that after the age of 70, most Indians will have slowed down or stopped their sex lives. Which is why when a 77-year-old patient of mine (I am not going to name him) asked me when he could resume his sex life, it took me a little by surprise, especially since he happened to be a widower.

When can you resume sexual activity?

Sexual activity can be safely resumed in about four weeks following an uncomplicated heart attack or angioplasty. Of course, the term 'uncomplicated heart attack' itself sounds like a paradox, but it indicates that the person did not have any other organ failure or prolonged stay in the ICU or need to be put on a ventilator. After an open heart surgery, it is safe to wait for six to eight weeks after the operation to allow the chest bone (sternum) to heal completely. Research has shown that patients who are exercising in a structured cardiac rehabilitation program have a better exercise capacity and this is associated with a lower risk of angina during sexual activity. *Angina d'amour* is the French phrase for angina that occurs during or immediately after sexual activity, and it is rare in patients who otherwise do not experience angina on exertion.

After a heart event it is quite normal to experience a drop in sexual desire, which may also be associated with a little bit of depression. Some patients may even experience erectile dysfunction, which they often describe as a loss of 'power'. There are drugs such as Viagra which are helpful in these cases, and they can be taken safely alongside most cardiac drugs. However, if you are taking a class of drugs known as nitrates (which are usually used for angina—such as sorbitrate), then you should not take Viagra. There is a possibility that this combination can lead to a sudden and dangerous fall of blood pressure.

In summary, sex is generally safe for those with heart disease, with a very low risk of untoward events. In fact, the only situation in which there is increased risk is when older men have been involved with younger women who are not their wives in an unfamiliar setting after excessive consumption of food and alcohol. This has actually been shown in studies, and the likely explanation is that the increased excitement associated with these unfamiliar situations puts an added strain on the heart.

Take-home messages

- After a cardiac event, it is safe to resume sexual activity when you can climb two flights of stairs without getting out of breath.

- As a general guideline, this will be a few weeks after an angioplasty, and six to eight weeks after bypass surgery.

- It is not safe to use erectile dysfunction medication (Viagra) if you are also on anti-anginal medication (nitrates).

19

How to Quit Smoking

(No butts about this)

ANIL SINGH IS A TOUGH NUT TO CRACK. LITERALLY. HE IS A RUGBY PLAYER, and is built and looks like one, complete with the shaven head. He is also the driving force and the founder of the Standard Chartered Mumbai Marathon, the largest and best-known marathon in India. I have known Anil well since 2003, and have had the privilege of being the Medical Director of the Mumbai Marathon since its inception until recently. Working with him has been fun, and we get on famously, except for one sore point. Anil is a smoker, and every opportunity I get I make sure I ask him to quit. I distinctly remember one conversation we had in Delhi, a day prior to the 2011 Delhi Half Marathon. It was at the pasta lunch for the elite athletes, and I took off on him one more time. He said, 'Docky, we all live only once and have to go some day. So why not enjoy our time on earth.' I agreed with his philosophy, which must have surprised him, but then added: 'It would be great if you could live exactly the way you wish, and then one fine day suddenly have a heart attack and drop dead. But what if you do not die? What if, instead of a heart attack, you have a stroke and are paralyzed for life, and live for another 20 years, with someone feeding you liquid food through a straw?' For the first time in my 10-year association with him, I saw the smile vanish from his face and he promised to give it serious thought. Well, that is one battle I have not yet won since Anil is back to his cigarettes, but I will continue to fight.

Easier said than done

If you've been a smoker for years, then quitting can be one of the hardest (if not the hardest) tasks you have ever attempted. When I lived in the US, my neighbour was a sweet 70-year-old lady, by the name of Sadie. Sadie had chronic lung disease, and needed to be on oxygen therapy permanently. This had made her homebound, and the only time she stepped out of her house was to shop for groceries or to visit her doctor, along with her portable oxygen cylinder. Her lung disease was caused by a lifetime of smoking, a habit which she could not quit. When I counselled her to give it up, she had tears in her eyes as she admitted that she had been trying for years, but was unable to do so. The addiction was so powerful she would need to smoke till late into the night. It was a sad sight to see her inhaling oxygen through prongs in her nose, and inhaling cigarette smoke simultaneously through her mouth. Eventually the smoking killed her, and when the end came, she had a pack of cigarettes beside her.

With the kind of information available today, there are very few smokers who say they do not want to quit. Most of them are desperate to knock off the habit, but are not able to. There are a few, though, who are still able to rationalize the habit, and efforts to get them to stop are destined to fail till the time they want to quit on their own. The reason why smoking is so hard to give up is the addictive effect of nicotine. As a drug it is as addictive as cocaine or heroin, the only difference being that it is legal. There is a physical and mental dependence on the drug, which is why most efforts at quitting tend to fail. After a few days of stopping, the physical withdrawal symptoms of nicotine set in, and they are so unpleasant that many will start smoking again just to get rid of these symptoms. Studies have shown that most people make several attempts at quitting before they finally succeed. The famous author Mark Twain was quoted as saying, 'Giving up smoking is the easiest thing in the world. I know because I've done it thousands of times.'

Benefits of quitting

It's never too late to quit smoking. It does not matter how long you've been smoking, the moment you quit your risk starts dropping. In fact, the benefits start from the minute you extinguish your last cigarette. Within the first hour your heart rate and blood pressure drop and the carbon monoxide level in your blood returns to normal. Over time your risk for heart attack, stroke and cancer starts dropping steadily towards that of a non-smoker. Of course, this information should not be used by you as a license to continue smoking with the thought that you will give it up one day in the future and recover all of your lost health. Remember, once there is build-up of plaque in your arteries, it can lead to a heart attack any time it ruptures. Smoking is one of the key factors that can precipitate plaque rupture, which is why even one cigarette can be harmful in the setting of blockages. It's similar to standing on the edge of a cliff. Even a slight push may be enough to topple you over; in the same way, one cigarette may be the final straw that broke the camel's back (no, not the cigarette brand, Camel).

In addition to the obvious health benefits of quitting, there are other social and economic benefits too. Think about all the money you can save by not spending on cigarettes. This may not sound like much over a week, or even a year, but if you look at 10 years or more, then the amount can be substantial. Besides, if you are looking at it purely economically, then you should also think of all the extra healthcare costs you will save yourself.

Socially, smoking is getting more unacceptable by the day. There was a time when it was considered cool to smoke, but I think that time has long gone, and today it's decidedly uncool. In fact, thanks to good legislation, in most parts of the world today, including India, smoking is banned in public spaces. It's quite sad to look at groups of smokers huddled outside bars, especially in winter. They clearly don't look like they're enjoying themselves!

A common excuse smokers use to avoid quitting is weight gain. It is true that most smokers gain some weight after quitting, but on an average, this is about 4-5 kilos. Clearly the health benefits of stopping far outweigh the downside of putting on that much weight. In any case, a good exercise program is recommended as part of your effort to quit, and this will have the benefit of offsetting any gain in weight.

Methods of quitting

For those of you who have grown up watching Bollywood movies in the '70s and '80s, you would have come across many a scene in which the hero is able to give up a lifelong vice in a single instant. He will throw down his packet of cigarettes, or smash his bottle of alcohol, and will vociferously take an oath never to touch the evil again. In medical terms we call this sudden stop 'cold turkey'. The chance of success by this method is about 5 per cent, though that of the Bollywood hero is always 100 per cent! There are many who are convinced that this is the only way to do it, and there is nothing wrong in giving it a shot. Even if you do not succeed on your first, second or fifth attempt, remember that every failure is a stepping stone to success. However clichéd this may sound, it is true, especially in the area of smoking cessation.

Two-step approach to quitting

I would suggest a more graded response consisting of two steps, rather than going cold turkey. The first step is to truly make up your mind that you want to quit. It's easy to say that you want to quit, since that's the right thing to say, especially to your doctor. You may want to quit to make your parent, spouse, child, or doctor happy, but the chances of success are highest when you want to quit for yourself and not because others are telling you to.

Quit date

Once you have made this commitment, set up a 'quit date'. This is the first day of the rest of your life, where you will be smoke-free. It's always nice to set a date which is of significance to your life, such as your birthday or anniversary. However, if a significant day is more than a couple of months away, then just pick a random date about four to six weeks from today. Once you select the date, go about telling the whole world. Often we never reveal our goals to others for fear that we'll fail, and people will know about it. This is the reason why I am suggesting precisely the opposite. By informing all those around you, you automatically set a higher standard for yourself and create an environment where it is more important for you to succeed.

Make a plan on gradually reducing your smoking from the day you decide till your quit date. For example, if you currently smoke 10 cigarettes a day, you can reduce your smoking by one cigarette a day every third day. In this manner, if your quit date is a month away, you will be down to zero on the selected date. As you approach the big day, start getting ready for a smoke-free life. Remove all cigarettes and associated articles such as ashtrays from your home, office, and car. If your social circle includes smokers, inform them of your decision, and ask them to support you. Vice loves company and it's often friends who smoke who may coax you back into the habit with comments like 'One won't hurt' or 'Let's have a smoke for old time's sake'.

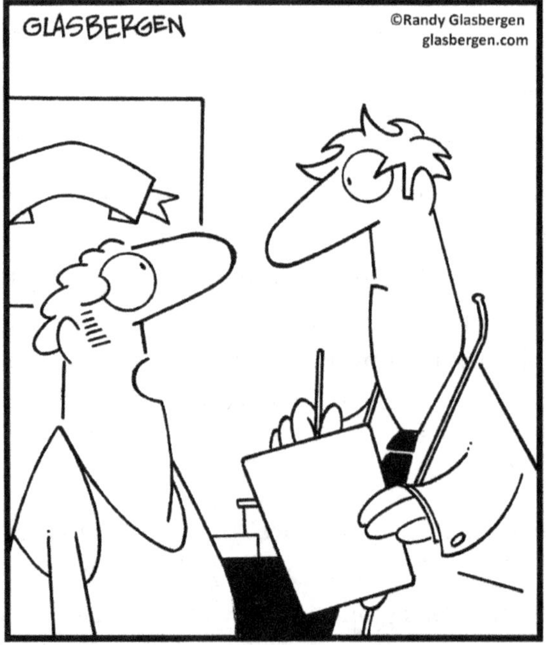

"I don't have time to jog or lift weights.
If it weren't for smoking, my lungs
wouldn't get any exercise at all!"

Nicotine replacement therapy

Since nicotine is the addictive substance in cigarette smoke, pharma companies came up with the idea of nicotine replacement therapy. The rationale behind it is to supply the body with small controlled doses of nicotine once a person has quit smoking. There are a number of methods through which this can be delivered, but the most common ones are the patch, gum, and lozenge. Ideally, you should start nicotine replacement right after you quit smoking for best chances of success. This will help you get through the symptoms of withdrawal, which include headaches, anxiety, irritability, and tiredness. There is no prescribed length of time for which it needs to be taken, but a two-month period should be good enough to help you transition to a nicotine-free life.

Recently, I saw a patient who lived in New York and had come for a consult since he got occasional chest pains. When I inquired about his smoking history, he told me he used to be a heavy smoker but had quit a year ago. I congratulated him, but he didn't look too happy, and explained the reason why. He had now gotten addicted to nicotine gum, and chewed over 20 a day! Clearly, the idea of using the gum is to transition towards freedom from nicotine and not the reverse.

E-cigarettes

I was at a party the other night and noticed something strange. There was a group of three well-heeled society ladies chatting together and smoking. That's not what was strange. What I found strange was that they were blowing out smoke rings, but I could not get the smell of cigarette smoke. My curiosity got the better of me, and I went up to one of them and asked about this anomaly. They shot me a look of pity, and said they were smoking e-cigarettes. I consider myself reasonably up to speed with the times, and have heard of e-mail, e-Bay, e-books, e-meetings, e-vites and even e-weddings, but what were e-cigarettes? I later found out that they were the latest rage on the party circuit, though they were originally touted as a means to quit smoking. E-cigarettes contain nicotine but do not contain tobacco. The nicotine is heated up and converted to vapour, which is inhaled and exhaled. At present there is very little data on their health effects, or on their usefulness as an aide to quit smoking. Until we have more information, I suggest you do not use them as nicotine replacement, and stick to gums and patches.

Other methods of quitting

One of my patients, a lifelong smoker, visited a hypnotist in London, and was cured of his addiction in one visit. Ordinarily I would be sceptical if someone told me such a story, but this was a first-hand account. Acupuncture, as well as other alternative therapies, have also been reported to help. However, none of these are scientifically proven, which is why it becomes difficult to recommend them. There are anti-smoking drugs which work by elevating your mood, which in turn will help you stay away from cigarettes. These have been shown to work in some people, but they do come with a few side effects.

In summary, there is no best method to help you quit, but for success, the most important ingredient is your desire to quit. This is one area of life where being called a quitter is a good thing.

Take-home messages

- ℗ Quitting smoking is very difficult, since nicotine is extremely addictive.

- ℗ However, it is the single best thing you can do for your health. Your risk for heart disease and cancer decreases steadily from the day you quit.

- ℗ Set a quit date and gradually reduce your smoking till you stop completely by that date.

- ℗ There are numerous aids in the market to help fight the addiction once you quit. Nicotine replacement therapy is the most popular of these.

20

Alternative Therapies

(Is there another way?)

'**D**OCTOR, I WANT TO AVOID BYPASS SURGERY AND TRY ALTERNATIVE therapy instead,' said Pascal Fernandes. He was a 53-year-old gentleman who used to work as the Chief Engineer on a merchant navy ship. He had an angio which revealed triple vessel disease, and was advised surgery. When I asked him what he meant by alternative therapy, he said he wanted to try lifestyle modification. This is a line I have heard very often, and it amuses me that people consider lifestyle changes to be alternative therapy. Wikipedia defines alternative therapy as any practice that is put forward as having the healing effects of medicine but is not based on evidence gathered using scientific methods. Actually, the preventive and curative effects of lifestyle changes have been very well documented, and should be considered as routine part of cardiac care and not as alternative therapy.

What is alternative therapy?

When used in the context of heart disease, most people view alternative therapy as any treatment apart from angioplasty and bypass surgery. However, do remember that lifestyle changes and risk factor reduction are the foundation you need to lay before considering any therapy. The most common of these alternative therapies is external counterpulsation (ECP), which is also commonly known as EECP, where the first letter stands for 'enhanced'.

How does ECP work?

When the heart contracts (systole), it pumps blood to the body, and when it relaxes (diastole), it receives blood. Diastole is also the time that the heart muscle (myocardium) receives blood from the coronary arteries. The principle behind ECP is an increase in blood supply to the myocardium during diastole. This is achieved by wrapping cuffs (which look like the cuffs placed around your arm to take blood pressure) around the leg in three locations. These cuffs inflate and deflate according to the rhythm of the heart, and push more blood to the heart during diastole. The treatment is usually done over 35 sittings, for an hour each. The goal of the therapy is to create collateral circulation by opening up smaller channels of blood.

How effective is it?

'Bypass the bypass surgery' is a catchy tagline you may have seen on billboards in centres across Mumbai. Many centres in Mumbai and across the country offer ECP as an 'alternative' to bypass surgery. In theory it seems like a credible option, as the function of the therapy is to create 'natural bypass channels'. However, there is no scientific evidence to indicate that ECP is an alternative to bypass surgery. It has been recommended for cases in which the patient has angina and has blockages which are not amenable to bypass surgery or angioplasty. In other words, it does have a valid role in selected cases, but it's important that the doctor place before you all the information that is required for making an informed choice. It would be wrong to recommend ECP as an alternative to bypass surgery in each and every case.

ECP is also useful in the setting of heart failure, where the pumping capacity of the heart is low. In my personal experience, several of these patients of heart failure do get an increase in their ejection fraction, though I should add that it does not happen in each and every patient.

Chelation therapy

Chelation therapy involves the intravenous infusion of a chemical called EDTA, along with other substances, over 30 sessions or more. The principle is that this cocktail of chemicals will bind and remove the calcium deposits in your arteries. These are then removed from the body via the kidneys.

Chelation was originally used in cases of lead and mercury poisoning. Each treatment session consists of giving these drugs via IV drip over a three to four hour period. This therapy has been practiced for a long time, but has always been regarded as controversial, and potentially harmful. At the end of 2012, a study carried out in the US suggested that, in certain selected cases, there may be benefit. This study was a huge shot in the arm for proponents of the therapy. However, several leading cardiologists have questioned the methods used in the study as well as the findings. Still, the study has caused the medical establishment to take chelation therapy more seriously, and review its effectiveness and side effects more closely. However, at the present moment it's still a therapy which falls under the 'not recommended' category by major medical societies.

Nutritional remedies

There are several hundred nutritional wonder remedies touted by doctors, nutritionists, quacks, housewives, and almost every other person you know. While most of these are harmless (and probably useless), there are some which can actually cause harm. Please remember one simple truth—there are no wonder remedies. Most food items have health benefits, but often these are highly exaggerated and suddenly they acquire the status of super foods, and you will find them everywhere, including the cover of magazines. Of late there is an email doing the rounds which talks about the wonders of pomegranate seeds. It claims that these seeds, when consumed in a particular manner, will not only help you get rid of angina, but will also 'dissolve' the blockages in your arteries. Pomegranates, like most fruits, are very healthy to consume. However, there is no evidence to back the tall claim that it can actually dissolve your blockages. This is a classic example of a good product around which false promises are woven. The internet is flooded with such 'wonder cures' for heart disease. One sure shot way of judging the authenticity of an internet site is to see if it's also selling the product for which it is making these claims. If it is, then I would view the information with more than a pinch of salt (which in turn will be bad for your blood pressure)!

Garlic is another food which is touted as a wonder food, especially to lower your blood pressure and cholesterol. Studies on garlic have shown equivocal results, with some of them showing reduction in cholesterol and blood pressure, and others showing no change. In any case, the studies in which garlic was shown to be effective had garlic consumed in very large quantities. If you had to eat that much garlic daily, I am not sure if your cholesterol will be any lower, but your friend circle might certainly decrease!

Ayurvedic and herbal medicine

This is a difficult topic for me to comment upon, since it's not my area of expertise. Ayurveda is an ancient medical science with many remedies which are very effective. The issue with a lot of indigenous systems of medicine is that they have not been through the same scientific scrutiny that 'Western' medicine has. That does not mean that they do not work, but it does mean that we do not have a specific basis to recommend them. As a rule of thumb, I would recommend that you do not stop your regular medications, especially life-saving ones such as aspirin. If you want to explore Ayurvedic therapies, make sure you consult with a senior practitioner and inform him or her about the allopathic medicines you are taking. The reverse is even more important. Often when patients meet their cardiologist, they hide the fact that they are taking other remedies for fear of upsetting their doctor. This is dangerous, since there is a risk of being over-treated for the same condition.

Acupuncture, faith-healing, and everything else

Heart disease is the world's largest killer, and therefore it's only natural that there are a wide range of remedies and solutions that claim to be curative. In my opinion, most of the more popular therapies may have some merit in them. Unfortunately, the claims they make are outrageous and end up discrediting the therapy, which otherwise may have been effective in a limited manner. The other danger of many unproven therapies is that they often encourage you to stop taking your routine cardiac medications, which may be a costly mistake.

Many patients will do anything to run away from conventional therapy. Remember the story of my patient, which I had described in the chapter on bypass surgery? He claimed that a 'baba' had put his hand through his chest, removed his heart, and repaired it by smearing some holy ash on it. He then put it back in the patient's chest, and all was well. Faith is often a double-edged sword. On the one hand, it's a powerful healer, and greatly aids a patient's recovery, and on the other, blind faith can lead to criminal neglect, especially when proven therapies are shunned in the name of faith. I think such cases should be defined as fate-healing, since the person is leaving himself to his fate rather than actively trying to get better.

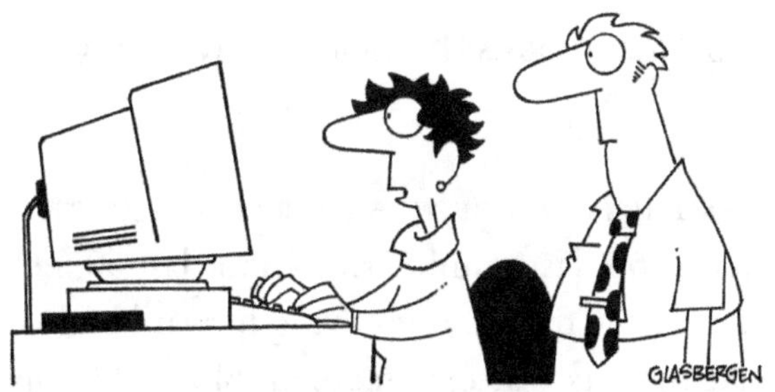

"I found 1837 web sites about 'alternative medicine' but none of them recommend pizza or chocolate for lowering our cholesterol."

Take-home messages

- ECP is a good therapy for some patients with angina and for patients with heart failure. However, it's not appropriate for every person with heart disease.

- Chelation therapy at present is not recommended for heart disease.

- Many alternative therapies have good effects, but often the claims made by those practicing them are greatly exaggerated.

- If you are taking alternative medications or nutritional supplements, make sure you inform your heart doctor about them.

21

Running Marathons after Heart Disease

(Distance makes the heart grow stronger)

IMAGINE THIS: IT'S THE FRIDAY BEFORE YOUR FIRST MARATHON ON SUNDAY, and you are out on your last training run. In the last 50 metres of the run, you hit an obstacle on the road and go flying forward and land directly on your face. To make matters worse, you are on blood-thinning medication, so the flow of blood doesn't stop. If that is not enough, you have asthma, and a history of epilepsy, which can make running hard. And to top it all, you have had open heart surgery two years ago and have never run after your school days. And did I mention, you are 68 years old! Before you cringe any further at my imagination, let me remind you that truth is indeed stranger than fiction, and such a person in flesh and blood (with a little loss of it) does exist and this unique individual is Surendra Dasadia.

Since its inception in 2004, every year, about 100 heart patients from the Cardiac Rehabilitation Centre at the Asian Heart Institute participate in the Standard Chartered Mumbai Marathon. Rather than call them heart patients, we should call them cardiac athletes. Seventy-five of these cardiac athletes run the 6-km Dream Run, and 25 of them run the 21.1-km half marathon. There is no better affirmation than this to prove to society that heart disease is not the end of life, but a new beginning.

Surendrabhai had done the Dream Run the previous year, and he came up to me in July and voiced his desire to run the half marathon. To be honest, I had mixed feelings about his participation. On the one hand, his enthusiasm was palpable and that to me is the most important ingredient in endurance training, but on the other, I was sceptical about his ability to go the distance, especially to run it. He had started jogging for the first time for a few hundred metres the previous month. To make matters complicated, he had an epileptic attack a few weeks later and had to be hospitalized for it. At this point I tried to dissuade him from participating and could see that he was clearly dejected. My heart went out to him, and we arrived at a compromise. We agreed to take it a week at a time, and take a final call closer to the end of the year.

In mid-September he joined our friend and chief motivator Mr Venkatraman (who is an inspiration himself) for outdoor runs at the MIG Club in Bandra. Surendrabhai was remarkably regular in his training, both at cardiac rehab, and with Venkat for the outdoor runs. Day by day he progressed, and by early January he looked ready and raring to go. On that fateful morning of Friday the 13th (of January), I got an SMS from Venkat informing me of Surendrabhai's fall, and both of us were very concerned. Surendrabhai was also very concerned—not about his injury, but about the fact that we may ask him not to participate! Once again he convinced me that he felt fit enough to run, and I relented. I am happy to tell you that not only did he participate, but he also finished in a very respectable time of 3 hours and 14 minutes.

Is there any health benefit to running marathons?

If exercise is beneficial for health, then more exercise should give more benefits, right? Actually, that's not the case. Research has shown that, beyond a point, you reach a plateau and there is no further health benefit. This plateau is seen anywhere between 2,000–3,500 calories expenditure per week in physical activity, which roughly translates to 30–50 km of walking or running per week. In fact, some studies have even shown some possible harm in 'over-exercising'. Let me hasten to add that this whole idea of excessive exercise being bad for you is a very new concept, with minimal data available at present. In any case, excessive in these cases are usually folks who engage in ultra-marathon training, and year after year are running in excess of 100 km per week. In general, these athletes are extremely healthy, but questions are being raised on the cardiac effects of such high volumes of training. In other words, there are certainly huge health benefits in running, but there may be no 'added' benefits in running very long distances.

Why then do people run marathons?

While pondering over this question, I was reminded of the classic answer Sir George Mallory gave when asked why he was so keen on climbing Mount Everest—'Because it's there.' The answer makes no sense to most people, but to anyone who has ever tried to achieve a difficult endurance goal, it's extremely easy to understand. Personally, I believe that running marathons is an activity undertaken by people for reasons other than health. It's done for a sense of achievement.

When running more than 20 km at a stretch, there is increased stress on your musculoskeletal system and it's debatable whether you get incremental health benefits by increasing mileage beyond a point. I have a confession to make. In spite of knowing this, I participate in endurance events and keep seeking to raise the bar. On April 1, 2012, along with my friends Jaideep Khanna and Prashant Mehta, I cycled from Mumbai to Pune and back, without stopping in between (except to attend nature's call). We covered a total of 329 km in 13 hours and 9 minutes. The real achievement was not so much the ride, but the fact that we raised over 1.2 crore rupees for St. Jude's Childcare Centre, an NGO which works with children suffering from cancer. The smile on the children's faces as we crossed the line made every bit of the effort worth it.

If you do want to set some big goals for yourself, by all means do so, but it's vital to understand your body and know the difference between achievement and harm. If you have had heart disease, then it's important that you discuss these goals in detail with your doctor and chalk out a sensible plan to achieve them.

How do I get started?

Most people who exercise do so through walking. In our country it is not very common to see people running, even young people. The first step to any successful running program is simple walking. Begin by walking for 30 minutes. Gradually increase the pace and time until you are able to cover a distance of 5.5 to 6 km in an hour. Keep doing this until it feels easy.

Introduce jogging

When you are comfortable walking briskly and want to step up the pace, simply add in a few jogs of 100 metres into your 60-minute walk. Warm up by walking slowly, build into a brisk walk and then do the short jogs when you feel ready. Once you achieve this, let's call it running, rather than jogging.

Slowly increase the amount of time you run

As you get more accustomed to running, increase the running segments gradually. Eventually you should be able to run for 40 minutes continuously. Do not worry about the pace. Below is a sample six-week training schedule to help you run for 40 minutes. Follow this for five days, and rest for two days every week.

	WALK-RUN (5 CYCLES OF 8 MIN EACH)	TOTAL TIME
1st week	7 mins-1 min	40 mins
2nd week	6 mins-2 mins	40 mins
3rd week	4 mins-4 mins	40 mins
4th week	3 mins-5 mins	40 mins
5th week	2 mins-6 mins	40 mins
6th week	1 min-7 mins	40 mins

Taking the next step

After you are capable of running for 40 minutes at a stretch, start focusing on distance. Work towards covering a distance of 5 km, which, depending on your speed, could range anywhere between 30-45 minutes. Once you are able to do that comfortably a few times a week for a few months, you are ready to take the next big step. Long-distance running is based on the foundation of long runs. Well, that does not sound exactly like rocket science, and it isn't. One day of the week, typically on the weekend, should be designated as your 'long run day'. On that day, you need to progressively run longer distances, increasing the mileage by about 5-10 per cent every week. The good news is that, on the other days of the week, shorter distances are just fine. In fact, you should not go for long runs more than once a week, especially as a beginner. A long run can be considered a distance of 10 km or more. Below is a 12-week sample training schedule for a half marathon. This schedule assumes that at baseline you are able to run comfortably for 5 km a few times a week. 'R' stands for rest, and is as important a part of your training as your running. Make sure you rest at least two days a week. Once a week, it's a good idea to cross-train, which refers to any cardiovascular exercise besides running. Cycling, swimming and elliptical training in the gym are good examples. In addition, though I have not included it in the table, you should do some light strength training at least one day a week, preferably two. This could be on the days you are running a shorter distance or cross-training. Your long run can be done on Sunday, if that's more convenient for you.

Are you allowed to walk in a marathon?

This is a question I often get asked, and the answer is, yes. There is no rule against walking in a marathon, but having said that, it's important to remember that the spirit of the race is to run. Your goal should be to train to run the distance, and add walking breaks as necessary. I would recommend that you plan these breaks, rather than be 'forced' to walk. Have a pre-planned run-to-walk ratio which you maintain throughout the race. It's best to plan it using time rather than distance. For example, you could decide to walk for a minute after every four minutes of running.

12-week half-marathon training plan

(All distances are in km)

Week	Sun	Mon	Tue	Wed	Thu	Fri	Sat
1	R	5	R	6	Cross- train (45 mins)	R	7
2	R	5	R	6	Cross- train (45 mins)	R	8
3	R	5	R	6	Cross- train (45 mins)	R	10
4	R	5	R	6	Cross- train (60 mins)	R	12
5	R	5	R	6	Cross- train (60 mins)	R	12
6	R	5	R	8	Cross- train (60 mins)	R	14
7	R	6	R	8	Cross- train (60 mins)	R	10
8	R	6	R	8	Cross- train (60 mins)	R	16
9	R	6	R	10	Cross- train (60 mins)	R	16
10	R	6	R	10	Cross- train (60 mins)	R	18
11	R	6	R	10	Cross- train (60 mins)	R	18
12	R	6	R	10	Cross- train (60 mins)	R	21.1

Safety first

Before you get into long distance training, it's necessary to get yourself thoroughly evaluated. I would suggest doing a stress echo test, which will give you an idea about your cardiac status as well as your current fitness level. While exercising, you need to take the usual precautions, as discussed in the chapter on exercise. You need to be particularly watchful, since you will be pushing yourself harder than before, and sometimes in the thrill of training, it's easy to get carried away. 'Listen to your body' is an old cliché, but is very applicable as you take this big leap forward. Again, I would like to stress that you must have a detailed discussion with your doctor before embarking on this journey. You may be on medication which affects your heart rate (beta blockers) and may need to adjust your training accordingly.

Hydration while running is another area to which you must pay attention, especially when you run outdoors in our hot and humid conditions. Earlier, we used to recommend that runners try and take in as much fluid as possible, but now we have realized that might not be the best approach. Instead, you need to balance your fluid intake with fluid loss. Your sweat rate is the amount of fluid you lose as sweat in an hour of running, and varies widely between individuals. In a study conducted by YouTooCanRun, it was found that sweat rates vary between half a litre per hour, to 2.5 litres per hour! You should calculate your sweat rate and take in the right amount fluid every 15 minutes during a long run to replenish the losses. For more information on how to do this, you can visit www.youtoocanrun.com, which has a sweat rate calculator as well as lots of other useful information for the cardiac athlete. Yes, you are an athlete and a star!

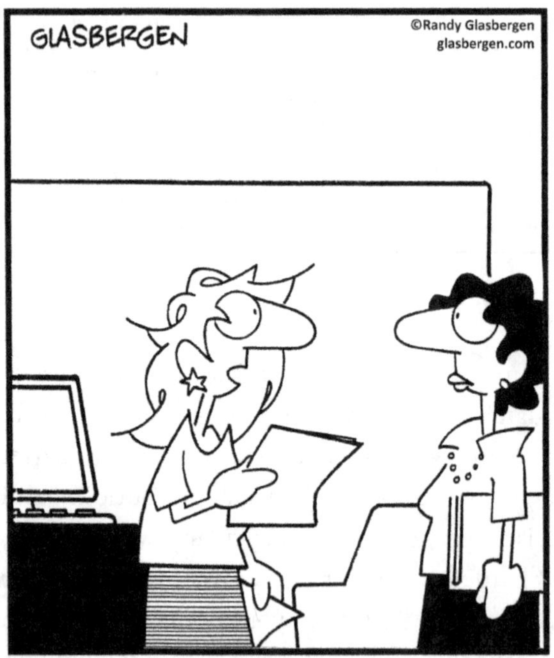

"I'm trying to squeeze 30 minutes
of exercise into my daily schedule.
Today I took 120 fifteen-second walks."

What a way to finish!

Now that you are a cardiac athlete, it's important that you keep up the momentum and your commitment to a healthy lifestyle. At the same time, you need to remember that just because you exercise regularly, you cannot ignore all the other aspects of care that we have discussed in the book. For the moment, though, enjoy the satisfaction of completing your first marathon.

Take-home messages

- You don't have to run marathons to get the health benefits of exercise. They are run more for a sense of achievement.

- Talk to your doctor before embarking on an endurance training program.

- Begin by walking briskly and then slowly adding short runs in between. Gradually increase the amount of time you run.

- When training for a marathon, you need to run long distances (more than 10 km) once a week.

- Safety is paramount, and you should be thoroughly evaluated before running a marathon, especially if you have heart disease.

$$22$$

The Book in a Chapter
(Putting it all together)

THE BOOK STARTED WITH A BRAVEHEART COMPLETING A MARATHON AND ended with a chapter on how you too can run a marathon. Between these pages, I have attempted to take you on a journey through the heart and empower you with the knowledge needed to prevent and reverse heart disease. I have tried to be as comprehensive as possible with the hope that complete understanding of the subject will enable you to better address this deadly killer. However, I do appreciate that not everyone may have the time or patience to read through every page. In the age of SMS and Twitter, even politicians now communicate in 140 characters or less, instead of longwinded speeches. Keeping that in mind, I decided to encapsulate the book in a chapter. For those faithful readers who have accompanied me through the journey, I hope this serves as a dessert after a fulfilling meal, and for those who just want to read this chapter, I hope it acts as an appetizer and tempts you to read the full book.

Working of the heart and the problems it can suffer

The heart has been considered the most important organ of the body since time immemorial and has received attention that is, frankly, disproportionate to the work it does. It simply acts as a muscular pump whose job it is to receive blood and then pump it out. Really, that's all it does! Impure blood from all over the body enters the right side of the heart, from where it is transported to the lungs. In the lungs, the blood gets purified and is returned to the left side of the heart, from where it is pumped to the entire body.

If you think of the heart as a house, it becomes easy to understand its structure, function, as well as the problems it suffers. Like a house, it has different rooms, two on the top (known as atria) and two at the bottom (known as ventricles). Like a house, it can have structural, mechanical, electrical and plumbing problems. Sometimes there is an opening in the wall between the left and right side of the heart, and this 'structural' problem leads to the mixing of pure and impure blood. This is usually a birth defect and commonly referred to as a hole in the heart.

The flow of blood in the heart is maintained in one direction due to the presence of valves. Sometimes there is a 'mechanical' problem and the valves don't open and close efficiently, leading to reduced flow or backflow of blood.

For the smooth and rhythmic contractions of the heart muscle, the electrical conduction pathways in the heart need to be functioning optimally. If not, there are rhythm problems which are felt as palpitations or irregular heart beats.

When I said that all the heart does is act as a muscular pump, I should have mentioned that it is probably the most efficient pump in the world. For an average human being, it does this three thousand million times from birth to death. To be able to do this, the heart muscle requires blood supply too, to keep it functioning. The blood vessels that supply blood to the heart are known as coronary arteries and run on the outer surface of the heart. There are three important ones: the left anterior descending (LAD) artery, the left circumflex artery and the right coronary artery. When there is a blockage in one of these, we can call it a 'plumbing' problem.

What we refer to as a plumbing problem is actually the largest killer of human beings today. These blockages are technically referred to as atherosclerosis, a Greek word which literally means hardening of the arteries. Since it occurs in the coronary arteries, it's also called coronary artery disease or coronary heart disease, and it leads to heart attacks. In the normal course of conversation, when we talk about heart disease we are actually referring to coronary artery disease, though all the other problems we discussed are also different aspects of heart disease.

Whilst heart disease is the leading cause of death for both men and women, the good news is that it is largely preventable. To prevent any illness we need to know what causes it, and these causes are known as risk factors. This is an important concept to grasp since it will help answer a lot of questions when coming to terms with why some people suffer and others don't. Think of the example of driving a car. Factors such as talking on your phone, or brakes not working well, drinking and driving, over-speeding, or an oil-spill on the road—all of these increase the chances of an accident, and these are risk factors. Clearly, the more of these that are present, the greater the chances of an accident. However, it is possible that none of these factors are present and you may yet have an accident; and, conversely, several of these factors may be present and you may still escape having an accident. It is very similar in the case of heart disease. Everyone knows of individuals who have lead high-risk lives and have been hale and hearty till a ripe old age, and we all know of someone close to us who lead a perfect and disciplined life and still had a heart attack at 45. Please remember that both of these are exceptions to the rule and make up less than 10 per cent of the population. In general, the more risk factors you have, the higher your chance of having a heart attack and vice-versa.

What are these risk factors?

Risk factors for heart disease can be broadly divided into two categories: those which can be modified and those which cannot. The non-modifiable risk factors are age and family history. Much as we hate to admit it, age is a one-way street. The older we get, the higher the risk for most chronic health ailments, heart disease included. In a Western population, the age cut-off is 45 years for men and 55 for women. It is higher for women since they are thought to be protected by female hormones prior to menopause, after which the risk is equal. In an Indian population, the risk is thought to begin almost a decade earlier.

Besides age, family history is something we cannot change. If your parents or siblings have had heart disease, your risk for the same goes up. It does not mean it's a fait accompli and that you *will* suffer, it just means that your risk is higher than someone who does not have a family history of heart disease.

Risk factors that can be modified are the usual suspects which most of us are familiar with. The big four are smoking, high blood pressure, diabetes and high cholesterol. In addition, lifestyle factors such as lack of exercise, unhealthy eating, obesity and high levels of stress are also risk factors which can and should be modified.

The more risk factors you have, the higher the chances of having heart disease. Often, those who end up having a heart attack are people who have several risk factors which are borderline rather than just one that may be very high. The danger of borderline values is that they tend to be ignored. It's also important to remember that just because your lifestyle may be healthy, it is not necessary that your risk factors will automatically be under control. In the recent past, a young and fit cricketer in Mumbai passed away in his early 40s, which understandably caused great worry among all those who read about it. Most people are unable to fathom how a fit person can get a heart attack. Unfortunately, fitness does not confer immunity against heart disease. It certainly lowers the risk, but it does not mean that a fit person will not suffer. In the example I cited earlier, it's akin to saying that a car cannot have an accident if its brakes are working fine. Functioning brakes are certainly important to avoid an accident, but it does not render you immune against one. Newer risk factors are being researched and discovered every year, but these are the most established ones as of today.

What is a heart attack?

The process of atherosclerosis usually takes place over several years and sometimes decades. The blockage, which is scientifically called 'plaque', grows steadily over time. Our earlier thinking was that this blockage kept growing until it cut off all blood supply within the artery and lead to a heart attack. We now know that this is not the case. At some point the plaque cracks or ruptures, and when this happens a clot is formed around the area, which shuts off blood flowing through the artery. This in turn leads to death of the heart muscle in the region supplied by that particular artery. This is called a myocardial infarction (MI) or heart attack. It's not necessarily the largest blockage which ruptures, which is why a 60 per cent blockage that ruptures is more dangerous than a 90 per cent blockage that is 'stable'.

Though we often use the phrase 'sudden heart attack', the actual process takes place over a long period of time and only the final event may be sudden.

Warning signs and symptoms

Most people consider chest pain on their left as a warning signal for heart problems known as angina. While this is the classic presentation of angina, in reality it may present itself in a variety of different ways. To keep it simple, remember that any discomfort from navel to nose could be related to your heart. The discomfort may present itself as pain, squeezing, burning, pressure or heaviness, and is usually related to exertion; that is, it increases with walking or running and reduces with rest. Discomfort that is due to gas or other digestive and muscular problems may also sometimes present in this manner, so when in doubt always get it checked out. If you feel these symptoms with a high degree of severity, then you may actually be experiencing an ongoing heart attack. Patients often describe it as 'an elephant sitting on their chest'. In such a situation, every minute counts, so make sure that you are taken to the nearest hospital in the shortest possible time. The best immediate treatment you can do is to chew on a tablet of aspirin en route to the hospital.

Making the diagnosis

'He had a complete check-up only a month ago and everything was all right, and still he had a heart attack.' As a doctor, I have heard this unfortunate statement many times, and it's a reflection of the fact that medical science still has a long way to go. To be honest, there is no perfect test that gives us all the information we need to diagnose and treat heart disease. Each test has its strengths and weaknesses and only a combination of tests, along with clinical history, will help give a complete picture. Of course, the final and most important ingredient is the doctor's own clinical experience and judgement in making a diagnosis and treatment plan based on the diagnosis.

Different kinds of tests

Some tests look at the functioning of the heart, while others look at the anatomy. Any type of stress test (such as stress echo or stress thallium) checks the functioning of the heart by looking at how the heart responds to stress (exercise) compared to rest. Other tests such as an angiography or CT angiography look at the anatomy of the coronary arteries to detect the presence of blockages. An ECG gives you a picture of the electrical conduction system of the heart and can help detect an ongoing heart attack, while a 2-D echo is done to check the pumping action of the heart along with the valve functions. Again, I must emphasize that there is no one 'best' or 'complete' test, and none of these tests should be performed as a matter of routine without your doctor prescribing it for you.

Options after diagnosis

Nobody likes to be told they have heart disease. And many don't like to admit it even if they do have it. I have come across many patients who have undergone bypass surgery, but if you ask if they have heart disease, they will deny it. Their logic is that the bypass was done purely as a preventive measure. To put it simply, anyone with proven blockages in their coronary arteries can be said to have heart disease. This is most accurately diagnosed with an angiogram.

Once this diagnosis is made, the all-important question is 'What next?' Broadly speaking there are two options: medical management or an intervention. An intervention refers to an angioplasty (also called PTCA) or a bypass surgery (CABG). Medical management refers to taking care of the patient without either of these interventions. It goes without saying that a program of appropriate lifestyle modification with a focus on exercise, nutrition and stress reduction is mandatory whether one undergoes an intervention or not. It therefore amuses (and sometimes angers) me when I hear people say that they do not want to do a surgery but instead pursue an 'alternative medicine' route of lifestyle changes. As I mentioned, lifestyle changes are the bedrock on which all treatment rests; it should not be viewed as an alternative approach.

Bypass surgery

Imagine you are driving down a highway when you suddenly come across a large construction zone due to which the road can continue no further. Invariably you will see a large orange sign saying 'detour' and will take the alternate route. Ultimately the alternate route will take you back to the original highway and the normal flow of traffic will continue. In many ways the principle of bypass surgery is similar. The surgeon 'bypasses' the blockage by connecting or grafting another artery below the region of the blockage. In other words, the blockage is bypassed and blood supply is restored via another artery, known as a bypass graft. The most commonly-used artery for this is your chest artery on the left side, known as LIMA (left internal mammary artery). Usually, one can be home within a week of the surgery, and gradual physical activity can and should be resumed once home. In fact, within two months of the surgery the patient should be better than before and not just back to normal, since 'normal' was probably not very healthy in the first place!

Angioplasty

In this procedure, which is also referred to as a PTCA, a catheter is passed through to the coronary arteries via the groin or the wrist, and a balloon is inflated at very high pressure to push the blockage to the sides of the artery. Invariably, but not always, a stent is then placed at the site of the blockage. The stent is a small cylindrical metal mesh which acts as a scaffolding to keep the artery open for a long period of time. Most stents today are coated with special medication to keep them open or 'patent' for a longer period of time. A person is usually discharged within 48 hours after the procedure is done.

Medical management

In fact, the most common option after being diagnosed with heart disease after an angiography is medical management. People like to simplify it by saying that the cardiologist advised them to 'do nothing'. Of course, this is misreading the advice because the cardiologist does not literally mean that you do nothing. It just means that an invasive procedure like angioplasty or surgery is not needed. What is needed is aggressive lifestyle modification along with optimal medication. Often, in such cases, patients tend to take matters very lightly since they feel that their situation is not serious enough to need an intervention. This is a dangerous trap to fall into, and one which you must be careful of.

Reversal of heart disease

Many books have been written on the subject of reversal of heart disease, but the concept is still confusing. The reason for this is that most people assume that reversal means that the blockages just shrink or maybe even disappear. That is not the case. What does happen is that the blockages become stabilized and do not rupture and lead to a heart attack. For practical purposes, that is what matters the most—in other words, it would be correct to say that 'physiological' reversal does take place, though it might not be 'anatomical' reversal. I have explained this concept in greater detail in the chapter on reversal.

For this reversal to take place, it is important to focus on the three important pillars of lifestyle: exercise, nutrition, and stress management. To be honest, in the information age that we live in today, most people know what the 'right' things to do are, but for various reasons they are not able to implement them. In the process, many tend to follow an all-or-nothing approach, which means they either do everything perfectly or not at all. It is very difficult to be on the right path all the time, both in life and lifestyle. My advice has always been to expect slips, and get back on track as soon as you can. If you can eat right and be physically active for most days in the year, then you have won the battle, even though there may be several 'off days'. One of the ways to approach this is to make simple rules for yourself which will help you stick to the program. These rules need to be relevant to your life and therefore cannot be generalized. I will give you a few examples which I have found to be useful as we talk more about the appropriate lifestyle you ought to be following.

Exercise

Many people get scared of the word exercise as they find it daunting. A gentler description would be physical activity, which is any body movement. Exercise is structured physical activity, and while they are similar, they are not the same. For example, if you walked from your home to the railway station for 10 minutes, it would be considered physical activity, but if it was a 30-minute walk and you did it briskly, you could consider it to be exercise. For heart disease prevention and reversal, both are important and often missing. My own parents are a classic example of the difference. My father is a very physically active person who is literally on his feet all day long. He belongs to the old school which still believes in largely travelling by the local bus, even though there is a car and driver waiting at home. However, he rarely does a structured exercise session. My mother, on the other hand, does not have much physical activity during the day though she is a doctor with a busy practice. But she exercises in a gym for at least four days a week for over an hour.

Which is better? That's a tough one to answer, especially since it will mean I am favouring one parent over the other, and that will get me into trouble! The easy and correct answer is that a combination of both would be the right choice. It's important to include a high amount of lifestyle physical activity, such as using the stairs instead of elevators, and at the same time participate in structured exercise at least three times a week for 30 minutes.

To simplify the exercise guidelines, here are easy-to-remember summary points:

- If you do not exercise currently, start by walking just 5 minutes daily. Each week, increase the time by five minutes till you are able to walk for 30-60 minutes at a brisk pace.
- Once you achieve this, you may increase the intensity by running, cycling, swimming or playing a sport. It's important to select an activity that you enjoy and will sustain. You can mix and match activities or continue only brisk walking if that's what you enjoy the most.
- Ideally, this structured exercise should be done at least three days a week for 30 minutes, while you should indulge in several short bouts of physical activity through the day. The goal is to slowly build up to 10,000 steps a day.
- Light resistance (weight) training is good to maintain muscle mass, especially as you age, and should be done two to three times per week.
- While exercising, if you feel uncomfortable in any way, stop and talk to your doctor before proceeding.

Nutrition

If there is one common factor which binds people across the world, it's our love for food. Along with this love come strong opinions on what does and does not make up a healthy diet. To make matters more confusing, the world of science and medicine is constantly changing and foods that were once considered evil are now considered good and vice-versa. It's almost like the fashion world, where styles are seen as 'in' or 'out' every few years.

Similarly, the advice on consumption of eggs, milk and shellfish, to name a few, keeps changing. In fact, even certain beliefs which we held as inviolable for long are now being questioned, such as the advice to keep fats to a minimum. To try and cut through the fat (no pun intended), I have come up with five dietary principles which will help you plan a healthful diet. Within these, I encourage you to create an individual meal plan which you will enjoy and sustain. So, here goes:

- 1:2:3 of diet—eat from all food groups: Imagine you are eating from a thali with six vatis. Select a mix of foods such that the approximate proportion is one portion of protein-rich foods, two portions of grains, and three portions of vegetables.

- Focus on fruits and vegetables: Eat a variety of fruits and vegetables, the more colourful the better. Also, remember that being 'vegetarian' is different from eating vegetables. The average Indian diet tends to be high in cereals and pulses and lacks in fruits and vegetables.

- Make it complex: While it's good to keep your life simple, it's better to make your food complex. Our diet tends to be very high in simple sugars, which end up being stored as excess weight as well as lead to a series of undesired metabolic consequences. Your diet should be high in complex carbohydrates and fibre, which helps reduce not only heart disease but also certain types of cancers.

- Watch the fat: Fat is the latest subject of controversy where diet is concerned, with several new studies showing that a very low-fat diet (which was once recommended for heart-disease prevention) is not necessary. To be honest, there are many types of fats which can be eaten in different proportions with differing effects on the body. In this summary, suffice it to say that fat content in the diet should be kept between 20–30 per cent, and saturated fat must be kept to a minimum. Trans fat, the kind found in some baked goods and biscuits to increase their shelf life, should be avoided completely.

- Size matters—calorie and weight control: Maintaining a healthy weight is key to good health. The goal should be to keep your BMI (body mass index) below 25 kg/m2. If it is more than that, you should aim to move towards that number through gradual weight loss of 1–2 kg per month. Where weight is concerned, it's largely a function of caloric balance. In other words, if we consume more calories than we burn, then we will put on weight. Towards that end, portion control during meals is extremely important, even when eating healthy food.

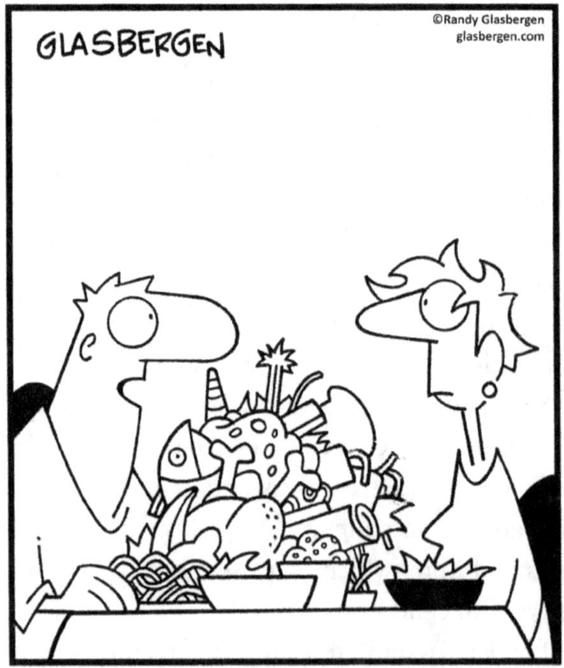

"If I follow 5 different diets at the same time, one of them is bound to work!"

Stress management

Most people attribute their heart disease largely to stress. Since we cannot measure stress in the same way we can measure weight or blood pressure or the other risk factors, it becomes very difficult to quantify. We know that stress contributes to heart disease, but it's difficult to say how much. Meditation is a great way to control your stress and should be practised on a regular basis. Yoga, which includes meditation and pranayama, is also an excellent method of stress control.

Putting it all together: life rules

Amitabh Khona never eats chocolates in India though he loves them. He only eats them when he is travelling abroad. While this may sound a bit strange, it's actually an interesting and effective rule he has made for himself to control his intake of sugar. Rajendra Jhaveri never eats rice at wedding functions since he suspects that they add extra oil to provide the soft, fluffy texture. Another patient of mine never went to the washroom on the same floor in his office complex. He always used the one on the floor above. Not because the one above was better or cleaner, it's just that it forced him to walk those extra steps daily.

All of the above are great examples of simple rules which can and should be incorporated into your daily life to help you adhere to the path of heart disease prevention and reversal. You need to make rules which fit into your lifestyle, because only then will you increase the chance of success. Bear in mind that you will often stray from the path, but the important thing is to steer yourself back as soon as possible. While this sounds a bit philosophical, it's true to life. The fight against heart disease is a long one, and you may be knocked down several times, but in the end it's not how many times you got knocked down that counts, but how many times you got up.

The heart truth

After 300-plus pages of reading, I hope that you have figured out the heart truth. To take care of the heart is not rocket science; rather, it's all about simple steps done consistently. Care really starts from childhood, during which time the foundation is laid for our future health. In many ways, the best care for the heart involves us going back to the days when we were children. Those were the times when we were active all day long, ate healthy, home-cooked meals, slept adequately and, most importantly, did not know the meaning of the word 'stress'. I assure you, if you are able to do all these, then you need not fear heart disease, and will remain forever young at heart.

23

Heart-Healthy Recipes

(Eating to your heart's content)

HEALTHY EATING HAS ALWAYS BEEN ASSOCIATED WITH FOOD THAT IS tasteless, but that should not be the case. Honestly, most of the best-tasting food in the world, made in traditional cooking styles, is also very heart-healthy. Often, a little tweaking of the usual cooking methods can increase the health quotient of your food. I requested two of India's best-known and loved chefs, Sanjeev Kapoor and Tarla Dalal (who has since passed away), to share a few of their recipes, in keeping with the nutrition guidelines we discussed. Bon appétit!

SANJEEV KAPOOR'S RECIPES

BREAKFAST

CHILLED WATERMELON AND CURD SMOOTHIE

Nutritive Value

Energy:	60.75 kcal
Protein:	2.7 gm
Carbohydrate:	9.98 gm
Fat:	1.08 gm
Fibre:	0.45 gm

Ingredients

½ cup seedless watermelon chunks
¼ cup low-fat curd
1 ice cube, crushed
¼ tbsp honey
1 tbsp chopped fresh mint

Method

- Freeze the watermelon chunks in the freezer for 3 to 4 hours.
- Blend the watermelon and curd with crushed ice and honey in a food processer.
- Stir in the mint leaves.
- Pour into a glass and serve chilled.

Palak Methi Thepla

Nutritive Value

Energy:	235 kcal
Protein:	7.6 gm
Carbohydrate:	34.6 gm
Fat:	7.3 gm
Fibre:	8.4 gm

Ingredients

¼ cup whole wheat flour
1 cup gram flour
1 tbsp shredded fresh spinach
1 tbsp chopped fresh fenugreek
A small pinch of turmeric powder
¼ tsp red chilli powder
¼ tsp ginger-green chilli paste
Salt to taste
½ + ½ tsp oil
1½ tbsp curd

Method

- Place the whole wheat flour, gram flour, spinach, fenugreek, turmeric powder, chilli powder, ginger-green chilli paste, salt and ½ teaspoon oil in a deep bowl and mix well.

- Add the curd and knead into semi-soft dough. Cover with a damp cloth and set aside for 15 minutes.
- Divide the dough into 3 equal portions and shape into balls. Roll out each ball into a 6-inch diameter thepla.
- Heat a non-stick tava. Place a thepla on it and cook turning sides and applying a little of the remaining oil on each side, till both the sides are evenly golden.
- Serve hot or cold.

SCRAMBLED EGG WITH MUSHROOMS AND PEAS

Nutritive Value

Energy: 192 kcal
Protein: 9 gm
Carbohydrate: 25.3 gm
Fat: 5.6 gm
Fibre: 4.3 gm

Ingredients

½ finely chopped large onion
2-3 fresh button mushrooms, sliced
1½ tbsp green peas, boiled
½ finely chopped large tomato
1 egg white, beaten well
½ tbsp chopped fresh coriander
A pinch of white pepper powder
Salt to taste
1 tsp oil
A slice of toasted multigrain bread

Method

- Heat the oil in a non-stick pan. Add the onions and sauté till they turn soft.
- Add the mushrooms and sprinkle some salt. Cook on high heat till the moisture dries up.
- Add the peas and tomato and sauté for a few seconds.
- Add the beaten egg white and stir continuously on medium heat till the egg scrambles. Add the chopped fresh coriander, salt and pepper.
- Mix well and serve immediately with toasted bread.

Lunch

Quick Jeera Chicken

Nutritive Value:

Energy: 263 kcal
Protein: 49.50 gm
Carbohydrate: 5.55 gm
Fat: 4.93 gm
Fibre: Negligible

Ingredients

¼ tsp cumin seeds
1 green chilli, sliced
½ medium onion, sliced
190 gms chicken on bone, without skin, cut into 1½ inch pieces
¼ tsp red chilli powder
A pinch of turmeric powder
Salt to taste
¼ tbsp lemon juice
½ tbsp chopped fresh coriander
1 tbsp hand-torn fresh mint
¼ tbsp oil

Method

- Heat the oil in a large shallow non-stick pan. Add the cumin seeds and sauté till they begin to change colour. Add the green chillies and onion and sauté till golden brown.
- Add the chicken and stir. Cover and cook, on medium heat, for 10 minutes.
- Add the red chilli powder, turmeric powder and salt and mix well. Cover again and cook for another 10 minutes or till the chicken is completely cooked.
- Add lemon juice, fresh coriander and mint and mix.
- Serve hot with rotis.

Dalia aur Dal Parantha

Nutritive Value

Energy: 308.5 kcal
Protein: 11.85 gm
Carbohydrate: 56.8 gm
Fat: 3.73 gm
Fibre: 9.68 gm

Ingredients

¼ cup dalia
1 tbsp whole green gram, soaked
¼ cup whole wheat flour
Salt to taste
¼ inch ginger, grated
⅛ cup finely chopped fresh coriander leaves
½ green chilli, finely chopped
½ tsp oil

Method

- Pressure-cook the dalia and whole green gram in ⅜ cup of water until soft. Cool and mash the mixture.
- Combine the wheat flour and salt. Add the cooked dalia and green gram, ginger, coriander leaves and green chilli. Add water, if required, a little at a time, and knead into soft and pliable dough. Keep the dough covered with a moist cloth for 15 minutes.
- Divide the dough into 2 equal portions and roll into balls. Roll out each portion into thin 5 to 6 inch diameter paranthas.
- Brush a little oil on a hot non-stick tava and place the parantha on it. Cook on medium heat for ½ a minute on each side. Reduce heat and cook further till both the sides are slightly browned.
- Serve hot.

Cucumber Pachdi

Nutritive Value

Energy: 39.5 kcal
Protein: 1.93 gm
Carbohydrate: 4.7 gm
Fat: 1.38 gm
Fibre: 1.3 gm

Ingredients

⅜ cup skimmed milk curd
½ small cucumber
¼ tsp finely chopped ginger
½ green chilli, finely chopped
Salt to taste
¼ tsp oil
⅛ tsp mustard seeds
2 curry leaves
½ dried red chilli, broken

Method

- Pour the skimmed milk curd into a clean muslin cloth and hang it for half an hour, preferably in a cool place.
- Wash and scrub the cucumber thoroughly and then grate with the skin.
- Pound together ginger and green chilli, in a mortar, to a fine paste.
- Mix the cucumber, ginger-green chilli paste and curd together. Add salt to taste.
- Heat oil in a small pan, add mustard seeds. When they start to splutter, add the curry leaves, red chillies and stir for a moment.
- Pour it over the curd mixture and mix well.
- Serve chilled.

DINNER

Chicken Parcels in Orange Sauce

Nutritive Value

Energy: 196.75 kcal
Protein: 33.7 gm

Carbohydrate: 4.68 gm
Fat: 4.85 gm
Fibre: 0.3 gm

Ingredients

1 medium chicken breast, skinned
¼ tbsp lemon juice
¼ tbsp Worcestershire sauce
¼ tsp mustard powder
A pinch of white pepper powder
Salt to taste
4 spinach leaves
¼ tbsp oil
¼ small onion, finely chopped
1 finely chopped garlic clove
20 gms low-fat paneer, grated

For the sauce

½ teaspoon corn flour
⅜ cup orange juice, preferably fresh
A dash of cinnamon powder
Salt to taste

Method

- Lightly flatten the chicken breast with a steak hammer. Retain the wing bone.
- Mix the lemon juice, Worcestershire sauce, mustard powder, white pepper powder and salt. Apply this marinade evenly on the chicken breast and leave in the refrigerator till required.
- Blanch the spinach leaves for 5 to 10 seconds in plenty of boiling water. Drain and cool.
- Heat the oil in a non-stick pan, add onion and garlic and sauté over high heat for 2 to 3 minutes or until the onion turns transluscent.
- Add the paneer and salt. Mix well and continue cooking for another 2 minutes, stirring continuously. Remove from heat and cool.
- Shape the paneer mixture into a ball.
- Place the blanched spinach leaves over the chicken to cover the entire top surface. Place the paneer ball on it. Place the breast on a 9 x 9 inch piece of

aluminium foil and gather into a bundle with the wing bone jutting out at the centre. Twist the ends of the foil around the bone to seal tightly, ensuring that the filling does not spill out.

- Boil sufficient water, reduce heat and poach the chicken roll, on medium heat, for 20 minutes or till done.
- Drain and remove the chicken roll, unwrap the aluminium foil and keep warm.

For the sauce

- Mix the corn flour and orange juice and bring to a boil in a non-stick pan, stirring continuously.
- Season with salt and cinnamon powder.

How to proceed

- Halve the chicken roll and serve with the orange sauce.

VEGETABLE CLEAR SOUP

Nutritive Value

Energy:	59.75 kcal
Protein:	2.4 gm
Carbohydrate:	8 gm
Fat:	2.08 gm
Fibre:	3.78 gm

Ingredients

1 garlic clove, sliced
1 mushroom, sliced
⅛ cup bean sprouts
¼ medium carrot, halved lengthwise and sliced
⅛ small cabbage, chopped into 1 cm pieces
¼ medium green capsicum, chopped into 1 cm pieces
4-5 spinach leaves, roughly chopped
1¼ cups vegetable stock or water
¼ medium tomato, seeded, chopped into 1 cm pieces
¼ tsp lemon juice
⅛ tsp crushed black peppercorns
⅛ tsp oil
Salt to taste

Method

- Heat the oil in a non-stick pan, add garlic and sauté for 30 seconds. Add mushroom, bean sprouts, carrot, cabbage, capsicum and spinach and stir.
- Add the vegetable stock or water and salt. Bring it to a boil and simmer for 2 minutes.
- Add the tomato, stir in the lemon juice and mix. Add crushed peppercorns.
- Serve hot.

VEGETABLE CRUDITÉS WITH CURD DIP

Nutritive Value

Energy:	135.25 kcal
Protein:	7.23 gm
Carbohydrate:	25.03 gm
Fat:	0.8 gm
Fibre:	7.38 gm

Ingredients

1 cup skimmed milk curd
4-5 fresh mint leaves
¼ tsp lemon juice
A pinch of toasted white sesame seeds
1 finely chopped garlic clove
2-3 iceberg lettuce leaves, soaked in chilled water
½ medium carrot, julienned
¼ medium white radish, julienned
1 red radish, quartered
½ medium cucumber, julienned
2-3 cherry tomatoes, halved
Salt to taste

Method

- Hang the curd in a muslin cloth to remove excess water.
- Reserve two mint leaves for decoration and chop the remaining.
- Combine the curd with chopped mint, lemon juice, sesame seeds and garlic and mix thoroughly. Add salt and chill.

- Just before serving, drain the lettuce leaves and spread on a serving plate. Arrange the cut vegetables decoratively on top of the lettuce leaves and serve with the chilled dip on the side.

RECIPES FROM TARLA DALAL

BREAKFAST MENU – 1

Carrot Coriander Juice	1 glass
Sprouted Moong and Methi Chila	3
Papaya	1 cup

Nutritive Value

Energy:	327 kcal
Protein:	14.8 gm
Carbohydrate:	50.4 gm
Fat:	7.1 gm
Fibre:	4.9 gm

CARROT CORIANDER JUICE

This juice is low in calories and is not strained so as to retain all the fibre in the juice.
Preparation time: 5 minutes
Cooking time: Nil
Serves 2

Ingredients

2 cups grated carrots
2 cups water
2 tbsp chopped coriander
½ tsp lemon juice
Salt to taste
8 ice cubes

Method

- Blend together the carrots and water in a mixer to get a smooth purée.
- Add the coriander, lemon juice and salt and serve over ice cubes.

SPROUTED MOONG DAL AND METHI CHILAS

Sprouts are a good source of protein, iron and Vitamin C, and a great add-on to our daily meals. This is an easy-to-make dish and ensures intake of sprouts for those who do not otherwise like them.

Preparation time: 10 minutes
Cooking time: 15 minutes
Makes 4 chilas

Ingredients

For the chilas

1 cup whole green gram sprouts
3 green chillies
1 inch piece ginger
½ cup fenugreek leaves, chopped
1 tbsp Bengal gram flour
Salt to taste
1 tsp oil for cooking

For the tempering

½ tsp cumin seeds
2 pinches asafoetida
1 tsp oil

To serve

4 tbsp low-fat curd, made from fat-free milk

Method

For the chilas

- Combine the green gram sprouts, green chillies, ginger and ½ cup water into a smooth batter.
- Add the fenugreek leaves, Bengal gram flour and salt and mix well. Keep aside.

For the tempering

- Heat the oil, add the cumin seeds and allow the seeds to crackle.
- Add the asafoetida and mix well.

How to proceed

- Pour the tempering over the batter and mix well.
- Heat and grease a non-stick tava with a little oil.
- Pour a ladleful of the batter on the tava and spread it evenly by moving the pan in a circular motion to make a 5-inch diameter chila.
- Drizzle a little oil on the sides and allow it to cook.
- When the chila is lightly browned, flip to the other side and cook again till it is golden brown in colour.
- Repeat to make 3 more chilas.
- Serve hot with low-fat curd.

BREAKFAST MENU – 2

Whole Wheat Hummus Wrap   **2**
Orange   **1 cup**

Nutritive Value

Energy:	308 kcal
Protein:	13.2 gm
Carbohydrate:	53.4 gm
Fat:	4.8 gm
Fibre:	3.9 gm

WHOLE WHEAT HUMMUS WRAP

The whole wheat salad wrap is rich in vitamin C, calcium, iron and fibre making a wholesome satiating snack from leftover chapattis. This dish can be put together quickly if the hummus has been prepared in advance and refrigerated.

Preparation time: 4 hours
Cooking time: 30 minutes
Makes 4 wraps

Ingredients

4 whole wheat chapatis, approx. 8 inches in diameter

For the hummus

½ cup chickpeas, soaked
1 tsp olive oil

1½ tsp garlic, chopped
Juice of 1 lemon
4 tbsp low-fat curd
Salt to taste
2 tsp tahini paste, recipe below

For the salad

½ cup tomatoes, thinly sliced
½ cup spring onions, sliced
½ cup carrot, cut into thin strips
1 cup lettuce, shredded
½ cup bean sprouts
2 tbsp finely chopped coriander
2 tbsp finely chopped mint
½ tsp roasted cumin powder
Juice of ½ lemon
1 tsp olive oil
Salt to taste

Method

For the hummus

- Soak the chickpeas in water for 6 hours making sure that they are covered with water.
- Cook the chickpeas in a pressure cooker. Cool and drain. Keep the drained liquid aside.
- Add the olive oil, garlic lemon juice, curd, cooked chickpeas, salt and some of the strained water from the chick peas in a blender and blend until smooth. If the mixture is too thick, add 2 to 3 tbsp of the reserved liquid.
- Keep refrigerated.

For the salad

- Combine all the vegetables, coriander and mint in a bowl and refrigerate for at least 30 minutes.
- Just before serving, add the cumin seed powder, lemon juice, olive oil and salt and mix well.

How to proceed

- Place one chapati on a clean dry surface.

- Spread an even layer of hummus on the chapati.
- Top with a generous portion of salad in the centre of the chapati and roll up tightly.
- Repeat to make the remaining 3 wraps.
- Serve immediately.

Tahini Paste

Tahini paste, which is an essential component of Lebanese cuisine, can be prepared within minutes by blending roasted sesame with other ingredients like lemon juice for a mellow citrus touch and garlic for lingering pungency. You need to take care while roasting the sesame because under-roasted sesame will have a raw smell while over-roasted sesame will become bitter. So, roast only till you get a strong aroma.

Preparation time: 2 minutes
Cooking time: 2 minutes
Makes 0.5 cup

Ingredients

2 tbsp sesame seeds
2 tbsp lemon juice
2 tbsp olive oil
½ tsp finely chopped garlic
Salt to taste
1 tbsp water

Method

- Roast the sesame seeds on a tava for a few seconds.
- Cool and then add all the remaining ingredients and blend in a mixer to a smooth paste.

Lunch Menu – 1

Makai Shorba	**1 serving**
Pyazwali Bhindi	**1 serving**
Chick Pea and Mint Rice	**1 serving**
Lauki ki Kheer	**1 serving**

Nutritive Value

Energy: 620 kcal
Protein: 18.4 gm
Carbohydrate: 85.2gm
Fat: 10.6 gm
Fibre: 9.0 gm

MAKAI SHORBA

Everyone is sure to relish this tempting Indian-style corn soup. This refreshing soup is a great energizer too. Serve hot with garlic bread to make an absolutely low-calorie 'hearty' meal.

Preparation time: 5 minutes
Cooking time: 12.5 minutes
Serves 2

Ingredients

2 cloves
1 inch cinnamon stick
2 peppercorns
1 bay leaf
¼ cup onions, chopped
2 cloves garlic, sliced
¼ cup carrots, cubed
½ teaspoon crushed coriander seeds
¼ teaspoon cumin powder
A pinch turmeric powder
½ cup sweet corn kernels
Salt to taste
1 tsp oil

To serve

Juice of a lemon
1 tbsp chopped coriander

Method

- Heat the oil in a pan, add the cloves, cinnamon, peppercorns, bay leaf, onions and garlic and cook till the onions are translucent.

- Add the carrots, coriander seeds, cumin powder and turmeric powder and cook for 3 to 4 minutes.
- Add the corn kernels, 3 cups of water and salt and simmer over a medium flame for 10 to 15 minutes till the corn is cooked.
- Cool completely and make a smooth purée in a blender. Transfer back into a pan.
- Bring to a boil and serve hot with the lemon juice and coriander.

Pyazwali Bhindi

A perfect, low-calorie version of the famous north Indian delicacy, in which the ladies finger is tossed with sautéed onions.

Traditionally the bhindi is deep-fried, but here is a heart-friendly variation to enjoy your favourite subzi and yet keep a check on calories as well as fat.

Preparation time: 15 minutes
Cooking time: 15 minutes
Serves 2

Ingredients

1 tsp cumin seeds
1 cup onions, chopped
2 tsp ginger-green chilli paste
A pinch of turmeric powder
2 cups chopped ladies finger
¼ cup low-fat curd
Salt to taste
2 tsp oil

Method

- Heat the oil in a non-stick pan, add the cumin seeds and allow them to crackle.
- Add the onions, ginger-green chilli paste, turmeric powder and cook till the onions turn golden brown.
- Add the ladies finger and cook over medium flame till they are soft.
- Add the curd and salt and cook for 2 to 3 more minutes.
- Serve hot with parathas.

Chickpea and Mint Rice

An all-rounder that contains ingredients from four food groups—cereals, pulses, veggies and oil, the Chickpea and Mint Rice is a satiating one-dish meal. The brown rice and mixed veggies used in this delicious preparation provide not just nutrients but also lots of fibre to keep cholesterol levels in check. All you need is to serve this quick and easy rice with a bowl of calcium-rich low-fat curd to make a balanced and complete meal.

Preparation time: 15 minutes
Cooking time: 5 minutes
Serves 4

Ingredients

1 tsp finely chopped garlic
½ cup thinly sliced onions
1 bay leaf
2 cups soaked and cooked brown rice
½ cup boiled chickpeas
½ cup chopped and boiled mixed vegetables (French beans, carrots and green peas)
Salt to taste
1 tsp green chilli paste
¼ cup finely chopped mint leaves
½ tsp lemon juice
1 tsp oil

Method

- Heat the oil in a broad non-stick pan, add the garlic, onions and bay leaf and sauté on a medium flame till the onions turn brown.
- Add the brown rice, kabuli chana, mixed vegetables and salt, mix well and cook on a medium flame for 1 to 2 minutes.
- Add the green chilli paste, mint leaves and lemon juice, mix well and cook on a medium flame for another minute.
- Serve hot.

Lauki ki Kheer

Everyone enjoys the traditional Indian kheer. Now try this traditional recipe in a healthy way to satisfy your sweet tooth. The recipe makes use of fibre-rich doodhi and low-fat milk and milk powder, which is easily available in all grocery stores.

Preparation time: 10 minutes
Cooking time: 20 minutes
Serves 4

Ingredients

1 cup grated bottle gourd
2 cups low-fat milk, 99.7% fat-free
2 tbsp sugar
½ tsp cardamom powder

Method

- Combine the bottle gourd and milk in a non-stick pan and simmer for 10 to 15 minutes till the bottle gourd is cooked.
- Add the sugar and cook till the sugar dissolves.
- Add the cardamom powder, mix well and refrigerate.
- Serve chilled.

Lunch Menu – 2

Garlic Vegetable Soup: 1 serving
Oriental Soya and Babycorn Stir-Fry: 3 servings
Oatmeal and Spinach Crépes: 2 crépes
Bulgur Wheat Salad: 1 serving
Apple: 1 serving

Nutritive Value

Energy:	615 kcal
Protein:	19.3 gm
Carbohydrate:	101.0 gm
Fat:	13.7 gm
Fibre:	8.1 gm

Garlic Vegetable Soup

A sumptuous soup of mixed vegetables flavoured predominantly with garlic, this nourishing recipe is innovatively thickened with rolled oats. This not only makes the soup creamy, but also adds more fibre to it.
Preparation time: 15 minutes
Cooking time: 15 minutes
Serves 4

Ingredients

2 tsp finely chopped garlic
¼ cup finely chopped onions
1 cup chopped and boiled mixed vegetables (French beans, carrots, green peas and cauliflower)
Salt and freshly ground black pepper to taste
2 tbsp quick-cooking rolled oats
2 tbsp chopped coriander
1 tsp oil

Method

- Heat the oil in a deep non-stick pan, add the garlic and onions and sauté on a medium flame for 1 to 2 minutes.
- Add the mixed vegetables, 3 cups of water, salt and pepper, mix well and cook on a medium flame for 2 minutes, while stirring occasionally.
- Add the oats and coriander
- Mix well and cook on a medium flame for another 1 minute.
- Serve hot.

Nutrient values per serving

Energy:	49 calories
Protein:	1.6 gm
Carbohydrate:	7.5 gm
Fat:	1.5 gm
Fibre:	1.2 gm

ORIENTAL SOYA AND BABYCORN STIR FRY

Stir-fries are always on top of the list when it comes to healthy cooking and monitoring the amount of fat used. In this recipe soya nuggets are chosen because of their ability to lower LDL (bad) cholesterol and baby corn to give the needed crunch without any amount of fat.

Preparation time: 10 minutes
Cooking time: 10 minutes
Serves 2

Ingredients

¼ cup soya nuggets
¼ cup spring onion whites, chopped
1 tsp garlic, chopped
½ cup mushrooms, sliced
½ cup babycorn, sliced and parboiled
¼ cup capsicum, diced
1 tsp soya sauce
2 tbsp tomato-chilli sauce
A pinch of sugar
Salt to taste
½ cup spring onion greens, chopped
1 tsp oil

Method

- Soak the soya nuggets in warm water for 10 to15 minutes. Drain and squeeze out the water.
- Heat the oil in a non-stick pan, add the spring onion whites and garlic and cook over high flame till the onions turn golden brown in colour.
- Add the mushrooms and cook till they are partially done.
- Add the soya nuggets, babycorn, capsicum and cook for 2 minutes.
- Add the soya sauce, tomato-chilli sauce, sugar and salt and cook for 2 minutes.
- Add the spring onion greens and cook for another 1 minute.
- Serve immediately.

OATMEAL AND SPINACH CRÊPES

These crêpes are made healthy by the use of whole wheat flour instead of maida. Oats and spinach have been added to further enrich them with fibre. In the filling too, cheese has been substituted with veggies, excluding the fat component.
Preparation time: 20 minutes
Cooking time: 25 minutes
Baking time: 20 minutes (Baking temperature: 230°C or 450°F)
Makes 8 crêpes

Ingredients

For the crêpes

2 cups chopped spinach
¾ cup whole wheat flour
¼ cup corn flour
3 tbsp quick-cooking rolled oats
1 tbsp oil
Salt to taste

For the stuffing

½ cup finely chopped zucchini
½ cup finely chopped brinjal
½ cup finely chopped capsicum
½ cup finely chopped onions
½ tsp finely chopped garlic
1 tbsp finely chopped celery
½ cup finely chopped tomatoes
½ tsp dried oregano
Salt and pepper to taste
1 tsp oil

For baking

2 ½ cups low-calorie white sauce, recipe below

For the low-calorie white sauce

1 ½ cups cauliflower or bottle gourd, chopped
1 tbsp butter
1 tbsp whole wheat flour
1 cup low-fat milk
Salt and pepper to taste

Method

For the low-calorie white sauce

- Boil the cauliflower or bottle gourd in 2 cups of water until soft. Blend in a liquidiser and strain.
- Heat the butter, add the whole wheat flour and sauté for a few seconds.

- Add the milk and cauliflower / bottle gourd purée and bring to a boil while stirring the mixture continuously till it becomes thick.
- Add salt and pepper and bring to a boil. Keep aside.
- *For the crêpes*
- Blanch the spinach in hot water for a few seconds and immerse in cold water.
- Drain and purée to a paste in a blender adding a little water if required.
- Mix together all the ingredients with enough water to make a batter of coating consistency.
- Heat a 6-inch diameter non-stick pan over medium flame and pour 3 tbsp of batter on the pan and move the pan in a circular motion, so as to spread the batter into a thin layer along the whole surface of the pan.
- Cook over a medium flame till the crêpe leaves the side of the pan. Remove and keep aside.
- Repeat with the remaining batter to make 7 more crêpes.

For the stuffing

- Heat the oil in a non-stick pan, add the zucchini, brinjal, capsicum, onions, garlic and celery and sauté for 2 minutes.
- Add the tomatoes and salt and cook for 5 to 7 minutes, till the vegetables are soft.
- Add the pepper and oregano and mix well. Allow it to cool.

How to proceed

- Spoon out 1 portion of the stuffing on to the centre of each pancake, spread a little white sauce on top and roll up.
- Arrange in a baking dish. Pour the remaining white sauce on top and bake in a hot oven at 230°C (450°F) for 20 minutes or until golden brown.
- Serve hot.

Dalia Salad

This is a simple yet different way of adding a nutritious cereal like bulgur wheat to your meals. Being loaded with high fibre and nutrient-dense veggies and dressed with a low-fat curd dressing, this salad is, by all means, one of the best-suited salads for people with heart disease or high blood cholesterol levels.

Preparation time: 15 minutes

No cooking

Serves 4

Ingredients

For the salad

½ cup dalia
¼ cup finely chopped carrots
¼ cup finely chopped tomatoes
¼ cup finely chopped capsicum
¼ cup mint, finely chopped
¼ cup chopped spring onion greens
½ tsp lemon juice
Salt to taste

For the dressing

½ cup low-fat curd, whisked
¼ teaspoon garlic paste
Salt to taste

Method

- Soak the dalia in water for 15 to 20 minutes. Drain and discard the water.
- Mix together all the ingredients.
- Mix all the ingredients for the dressing
- Toss the salad and dressing together lightly and serve immediately.

SNACK MENU – 1

Soya Poha: 1 serving
Apple: 1

Nutritive Value

Energy: 196 kcal
Protein: 8.4 gm
Carbohydrate: 20.1 gm
Fat: 5.3 gm
Fibre: 4.3 gm

Soya Poha

Soybeans are a powerhouse of nutrients. They are used here in granule form to whip up an appetizing version of poha, a popular Maharashtrian snack. Eat this unusual version regularly to benefit from the goodness of soya.

Preparation time: 5 minutes

Cooking time: 10 minutes

Serves 4

Ingredients

1¼ cups soya granules

1 tsp mustard seeds

1 tsp urad dal

5 to 6 curry leaves

¼ tsp asafoetida

½ cup sliced onions

1 tsp finely chopped green chillies

1 tbsp chopped coriander

¼ tsp turmeric powder

½ tsp chilli powder

¼ cup boiled green peas

2 tsp lemon juice

2 tsp oil

Salt to taste

For the garnish

2 tbsp chopped coriander

Method

- Soak the soya granules in 2 cups of warm water for 30 minutes. Squeeze and keep aside.
- Heat the oil in a non-stick pan and add the mustard seeds, urad dal, curry leaves and asafoetida and sauté till the seeds crackle.
- Add the onions and green chillies and sauté till the onions turn translucent.
- Add the coriander, turmeric powder, chilli powder and salt and mix well.
- Add the soya granules and green peas and sauté for another 3 to 4 minutes.
- Remove from the flame, add the lemon juice and mix well.
- Serve hot, garnished with coriander.

Snack Menu – 2

Creamy Alfa-Alfa Sprouts and Apple on Toast: 1 sandwich
Golden Glory Frappe: 1 serving

Nutritive Value

Energy: 230 kcal
Protein: 9.9 gm
Carbohydrate: 47.4 gm
Fat: 1.1 gm
Fibre: 3.0 gm

Creamy Alfa-Alfa Sprouts and Apple on Toast

In this sumptuous snack, whole wheat bread slices are topped with a healthy topping of low-fat curd, sprouts, apples, and other ingredients perked up with mustard powder and black pepper powder. While this recipe uses alfa-alfa sprouts, you can try a similar topping with bean sprouts too.

Preparation time: 10 minutes
Cooking time: Nil
Makes 2 toasts

Ingredients

2 toasted whole wheat bread slices
For the topping
¼ cup low-fat curd
½ cup alfa-alfa sprouts
¼ cup grated apples
1 tbsp finely chopped celery
2 tbsp chopped spring onion whites and greens
½ tsp mustard powder
Salt and freshly ground black pepper to taste

Method

- Mix all the ingredients for the topping together.
- Divide the topping into 2 equal portions and spread on each toast.
- Serve immediately.

GOLDEN GLORY FRAPPÉ

This cool, refreshing drink is appealing nutritionally as well as visually due to its colour. Nutmeg further adds a touch of flavour to this low-fat, high-fibre drink. The combination of sweet papaya and honey helps to avoid the use of sugar completely.

Preparation time: 5 minutes
Cooking time: Nil
Serves 2

Ingredients

1½ cups papaya pieces
½ cup apple pieces
¼ cup low-fat curd
A pinch nutmeg powder
1 tsp honey
6 to 8 ice cubes

Method

- Combine all the ingredients along with 1 cup water and purée till it is smooth.
- Pour into 2 glasses and serve immediately.

DINNER MENU – 1

Oat and Spring Onion Paratha: 1
Lauki Kofta Curry: 1 serving
Cabbage Pulao: 1 serving
Carrot and Mint Salad: 1 serving
Pineapple, chopped: 1 cup

Nutritive Value

Energy:	619 kcal
Protein:	19.8 gm
Carbohydrate:	116.7 gm
Fat:	8.7 gm
Fibre:	6.2 gm

OAT AND SPRING ONION PARATHAS

These parathas are made with a combination of oats and wheat flour to initiate you to the taste of fibre-filled oats. Spring onion filling helps to disguise the raw taste of oats. They taste best when served hot.

Preparation time: 15 minutes
Cooking time: 20 minutes
Makes 4 parathas

Ingredients

For the dough

¾ cup whole wheat flour
¼ cup quick-cooking rolled oats
2 tbsp curd
Salt to taste

For the spring onion filling

1 tsp cumin seeds
½ cup chopped spring onion whites
1 tsp ginger-green chilli paste
1 tsp finely chopped garlic
1 cup chopped spring onion greens
½ tsp oil
Salt to taste

Other ingredients

1 tsp oil for cooking

Method

For the dough

- Combine all the ingredients and knead into a soft dough, using enough water.
- Divide into 4 equal portions and keep aside.

For the filling

- Heat the oil in a pan, add the cumin seeds and allow the seeds to crackle.
- Add the spring onion whites, ginger-green chilli paste, garlic and cook till the onions turn translucent.

- Add the spring onion greens and salt and cook over a high flame till the mixture dries out completely. Remove and let it cool.

How to proceed

- Roll out each portion of the dough into a circle of 3 inches diameter.
- Place a portion of the filling in the centre of the dough circle.
- Bring together all the sides in the centre and seal tightly.
- Roll out again into a circle of 5 inches diameter with the help of a little plain flour.
- Cook the paratha on a non-stick pan, using a little oil, until both sides are golden brown.
- Repeat with the remaining dough and filling to make 3 more parathas.
- Serve hot.

Lauki Kofta Curry

These koftas are prepared with lauki in a larger proportion, in comparison to potato, to minimise the caloric value of the dish. Also, koftas are not deep-fried, but are simmered and cooked in the curry itself.

Preparation time: 15 minutes
Cooking time: 10 minutes
Serves 4

Ingredients

For the lauki koftas

1½ cups grated bottle gourd
⅓ cup boiled, peeled and mashed potatoes
½ cup Bengal gram flour
1½ tsp finely chopped green chillies
1 tsp ginger-garlic paste
1 tsp chaat masala
Salt to taste

For the curry

1 tsp oil
1 tsp cumin seeds
½ cup grated onions

1 tsp ginger paste
1 tsp garlic paste
½ cup grated tomatoes
½ tsp turmeric powder
½ tsp coriander-cumin seeds powder
½ tsp chilli powder
Salt to taste
1 tsp corn flour dissolved in 2 tbsp low-fat milk
½ tsp garam masala

Method

For the lauki koftas

- Strain the liquid out of the bottle gourd and preserve it to add in the gravy.
- Combine all the ingredients in a non-stick pan and stir it over medium flame till the mixture leaves the sides of the pan.
- Remove and cool slightly. Divide this mixture into 14 equal portions and roll each portion into oval koftas. Keep aside.

For the curry

- Heat the oil in a deep non-stick pan and add the cumin seeds.
- When the seeds crackle, add the onions and sauté on a medium flame for a minute.
- Add the ginger paste, garlic paste, tomatoes, turmeric powder, coriander-cumin seeds powder and chilli powder and cook for 1 to 2 minutes, while stirring occasionally.
- Add the reserved liquid of the bottle gourd and 1½ cups of water, mix well and bring to a boil, while stirring occasionally.
- Add the salt and corn flour-milk mixture, mix well and cook on a medium flame for 1 minute, while stirring occasionally.
- Add the koftas, and garam masala, mix gently and cook on a medium flame for another 1 to 2 minutes.
- Serve hot with parathas or brown rice.
- Tip: The koftas tend to crumble if you boil them too much in the gravy, so, it's better to add them just before you're ready to serve them.

CABBAGE PULAO

This is an easy to make rice delicacy, put together especially for fans of south Indian food. This recipe makes use of cabbage and a tempering of urad dal, both ingredients being most popular in south Indian cooking.

Preparation time: 10 minutes

Cooking time: 10 minutes

Serves 2

Ingredients

½ tsp mustard seeds

½ tsp split black lentils

A pinch asafoetida

4 to 5 curry leaves

3 dry red chillies, broken into 1inch pieces

¼ cup thinly sliced onions

A pinch of turmeric powder

1 cup shredded cabbage

¼ cup split Bengal gram, parboiled

1 cup boiled rice

½ tsp lemon juice

1 tsp oil

Salt to taste

For the garnish

1 tbsp chopped coriander

Method

- Heat the oil in a non-stick pan, add the mustard seeds and allow them to crackle.
- Add the split black lentils, asafoetida, curry leaves and dry red chillies and cook for 1 minute till the lentils turns pink.
- Add the onions and turmeric powder and cook for another 1 minute.
- Add the cabbage, split Bengal gram, salt and 1 tbsp water and cook over a low flame for 5 minutes or till the cabbage is tender.
- Add the rice and lemon juice, mix well and cook covered for a few minutes.
- Serve hot, garnished with coriander.

Carrot and Mint Salad

Carrots combined with cucumber, kidney beans and spring onions are laced with a minty dressing. This salad, served with Lauki Kofta Curry, and Oat and Spring Onion Paratha makes a complete and healthy meal.

Preparation time: 10 minutes
Cooking time: Nil
Serves 2

Ingredients

1 cup carrots, peeled and thinly sliced
1 cup cucumber, peeled and thinly sliced
½ cup kidney beans, boiled
½ cup spring onions, sliced

For the dressing

1 tbsp mint, finely chopped
1 tsp honey
1 tbsp lemon juice
Salt to taste

Method

- Combine all the ingredients for the salad in a bowl and chill.
- Combine all the elements for the dressing.
- Just before serving, add the dressing and toss well.
- Serve immediately.

Dinner Menu – 2

Spinach Soup with Garlic: 1 serving
Crunchy Cumin Seeds Crackers: 5
Sweet Potato Salad: 1 serving
Full of Fibre Pasta: 1 serving
Baked Cottage Cheese Pie: 1 serving
Papaya, Sliced: 1 cup

Nutritive Value

Energy: 624 kcal
Protein: 20.1 gm
Carbohydrate: 72.2 gm
Fat: 8.5 gm
Fibre: 8.6 gm

SPINACH SOUP WITH GARLIC

This nutritious, low-fat, low-calorie soup is best if you are trying to lose some of those extra pounds.

Preparation time: 15 minutes
Cooking time: 15 minutes
Serves 4

Ingredients

½ cup finely chopped onions
1 tbsp roughly chopped garlic
3 cups chopped spinach
1 tsp corn flour dissolved in ½ cup low-fat milk
Salt and freshly ground pepper to taste
1 tsp oil

For serving

Toasted whole wheat bread

Method

- Heat the oil in a non-stick pan, add the onions and garlic and sauté on a medium flame for 1 to 2 minutes.
- Add the spinach and cook on a medium flame for 2 minutes.
- Add 1 cup of cold water and purée the mixture in a blender to a coarse texture.
- Pour the purée back to the pan, add the corn flour-milk mixture, salt and pepper and bring to a boil.
- Serve hot with toasted whole wheat bread.

CRUNCHY CUMIN SEED CRACKERS

These crispy, low-fat munchies are made with oats, maize flour and whole-wheat flour instead of refined maida. These are great to keep in your handbag so that you are prepared when hunger strikes. You can also serve them as an appetiser along with garlic tomato salsa.

Preparation time: 10 minutes
Cooking time: Nil
Makes 20 crackers
Baking time: 40 minutes (Baking temperature: 160°C or 320°F)

Ingredients

¾ cup whole wheat flour
1½ tsp corn flour
2 tbsp maize flour
2 tsp low-fat milk (99.7% fat-free)
¼ cup quick-cooking rolled oats
½ tsp cumin seeds
1 tbsp low-fat curd
1 tbsp oil
Salt to taste

Other ingredients

1 tsp oil for greasing

Method

- Combine all the ingredients in a bowl, mix well and knead into a firm dough using enough water.
- Divide the dough into 20 equal portions and roll each portion to 2 mm thickness.
- Prick the dough with the help of a toothpick and cut into squares that are 50 mm (2 inches).
- Place on a greased baking tray and bake in a pre-heated oven for 30 minutes at 160°c (320°f) or until lightly brown and crisp.
- Cool and store in an air-tight container.
- Tip: The crackers will appear a little soft when hot, but will get crisp once they cool down to room temperature.

SWEET POTATO SALAD

Combine the starchy sweet potato with other vegetables to add fibre to your diet. Another addition to this wonderful salad is walnuts, which helps to strengthen the heart, and apples which lend the necessary sweetness while avoiding unnecessary calories from sugar.

Preparation time: 15 minutes

Cooking time: Nil

Serves 4

Ingredients

1 cup sweet potatoes, boiled and cut into 1-inch cubes
¾ cup apples, diced (unpeeled)
½ cup walnuts, chopped
½ cup celery, chopped
½ cup capsicum, cut into 1-inch cubes
1 tsp lemon juice

For the dressing

½ cup low-fat curd
½ teaspoon prepared mustard paste
Salt and pepper to taste

Method

- Mix all the ingredients for the salad together in a large bowl.
- Mix all the ingredients for the dressing together, add to the salad and refrigerate.
- Serve chilled.

FULL OF FIBRE PASTA

As the name suggests, this pasta is full of fibre. The use of whole wheat pasta and lots of vegetables is the specialty of this fibre-rich dish.

Preparation time: 10 minutes

Cooking time: 10 minutes

Serves 2

Ingredients

For the sauce

½ cup finely chopped onions
¼ cup boiled sweet corn kernels
¼ cup chopped capsicum

2 tsp finely chopped garlic
½ cup low-fat milk
1 tsp corn flour
1 tsp oil
Salt and freshly ground black pepper to taste

For the pasta

1 tsp finely chopped garlic
1 dry red chilli chopped
1½ cups cooked whole wheat pasta
½ tsp oil

For the garnish

1 tbsp finely chopped parsley

Method

For the sauce

- Heat the oil and add the onions.
- Sauté the onions over a low flame for 4 to 6 minutes till they are soft.
- Add the vegetables, garlic and salt and sauté again for 5 to 7 minutes.
- Add ¼ cup water and cover and simmer till the vegetables are soft.
- Add the milk and corn flour and mix well.
- Bring to a boil, add the pepper and keep aside.

For the pasta

- Heat the oil in a non-stick pan and add the garlic and red chilli and sauté for a few seconds.
- Add the pasta and toss well.
- Add the prepared sauce and mix well.
- Serve hot, topped with the parsley.
- Tip: You may use fusilli, penne or tagliatelle pasta.

BAKED APPLE COTTAGE CHEESE PIE

A dessert which tastes delicious when served warm. Made just with low-fat paneer and fruits, you can occasionally enjoy a serving of this dessert after your meal. However, do remember to include these calories as part of your diet.

Preparation time: 10 minutes
Baking time: 15 minutes (Baking temperature: 220°C or 440°F)
Serves 4

Ingredients

For the cottage cheese mixture

1 cup low-fat cottage cheese cubes
4 tsp sugar
A few strands of saffron dissolved in 4 tbsp low-fat milk (99.7% fat free)
1 tsp corn flour
A few strands of saffron strands

For the fruit filling

1 cup sliced apple
4 tsp brown sugar
¼ tsp nutmeg powder
A few drops lemon juice

Method

For the cottage cheese mixture

- Blend all the ingredients into a smooth mixture.

For the fruit filling

- Combine all the ingredients in a deep bowl, cover and keep aside for 15 minutes.
- Arrange the fruit in a greased 150 mm (6-inch) diameter pie dish.

How to proceed

- Spread the cottage cheese mixture over the fruit and bake in a pre-heated oven at 220°C (440°f) for 15 minutes.
- Serve warm.

Acknowledgements

I AM NOT a person who makes New Year resolutions, but I had resolved to run a half marathon in less than an hour and 45 minutes, and to write a book before my fortieth birthday. Well, I managed the former and am happy to say that the latter has come to fruition too, albeit four years late. Several people and institutions have helped build my experience base, which allowed me to write this book. Chief among them are my patients, who have helped me as much as I hope I have helped them. Through the book, I share their real-life experiences, along with their true identities, in most places.

Speaking of patients, I need to acknowledge the patience of my editor, Deepthi Talwar. She has been a great support through the whole process and was there to answer all the questions of a 'newbie' author.

I would like to acknowledge Dr Ramakanta Panda and the Asian Heart Institute, where I spent many happy years of my career.

Shashank Joshi has been a friend and a guide on many aspects of the book, and I would like to acknowledge his help.

Many thanks to Chef Sanjeev Kapoor and the late Tarla Dalal for contributing their heart-healthy recipes.

I am also most grateful to my family, for always being there in every way, whether it's cheering during a marathon, or writing a book.

9 789360 454876